SUZY PRUDDEN'S
I CAN EXERCISE ANYWHERE BOOK

**Books by Suzy Prudden and
Jeffrey Sussman**

Creative Fitness For Baby & Child
Suzy Prudden's Family Fitness Book
Fit For Life
See How They Run
Suzy Prudden's Spot Reducing Program
Suzy Prudden's Pregnancy & Back-to-Shape
   Exercise Program

SUZY PRUDDEN'S
I CAN EXERCISE ANYWHERE
BOOK

by Suzy Prudden & Jeffrey Sussman

Photographs by Nancy DePra

Workman Publishing, New York

DEDICATION

To the "2nd chance" and the Ettenbergs, the people connected to it. May our new friendship and program prosper and be as healthy and happy in the coming years as I am now.

And to two very special friends at the opposite ends of my generation gaps. My son, Robby Sussman, a close friend, who is blossoming into a wonderful, sensitive, thoughtful and joyous young man; and to a new, but dear old friend, my mother, Bonnie Prudden. Now my best friend. I can see beyond tomorrow; learn and accomplish anything because she taught me how.

—Suzy Prudden

For words said and deeds done. To my friends: Councilman Henry Stern, Frank Cogan, Steve Schwartz, Tom Damico and Tweetie.

—Jeffrey Sussman

Library of Congress Cataloging in Publication Data

Prudden, Suzy.
　Suzy Prudden's I can exercise anywhere book.

　1. Exercise.　I. Sussman, Jeffrey.　II. Title.
III. Title: I can exercise anywhere book.
RA781.P763　　613.7'1　　81-40507
ISBN 0-89480-185-6　　　　　　AACR2
ISBN 0-89480-186-4 (pbk.)

Cover and book design: Wendy Palitz

Suzy Prudden's leotards of nylon with Lycra spandex by Capezio Ballet Makers

Manufactured in the United States of America
First printing November 1981

10 9 8 7 6 5 4 3 2 1

Workman Publishing Company, Inc.
1 West 39 Street
New York, New York 10018

CONTENTS

INTRODUCTION

More and more people are keeping fit and trim these days. You see them in the gyms, on the jogging trails, all across the country. You hear about them on radio and television, in newspapers and magazines. You'd probably like to join them. But you simply don't have the time. You're a busy executive, a harassed housewife, a businessperson on the go, an overworked student. Your calendar is crammed with things to do. You're just too busy to keep fit.

Well, you've just run out of excuses.

Over the years, many people have asked us the same question: What can I do if I don't have the time to work out? The answer is remarkably simple. If you can't adjust your schedule to fit in any exercise, adjust the exercises so that they will fit into your schedule! We all experience wasted moments—standing on long lines, sitting in waiting rooms, traveling in cars, buses, or trains, on telephones after the operator has put you on hold for the third time. Many of the exercises in this book were designed to be used in those moments. There are other times when you could easily be doing two things at once—when you sit in front of the television, for example. We have provided routines to take care of those as well. If you combine a selection of these exercises with a brisk walk every day, you will have embarked on a complete, healthful exercise program that will keep you fit and trim—and that will hardly take up any time at all.

When you wake up in the morning, have you ever lain in bed for an extra five minutes after the alarm rings? Spend those minutes stretching your sleepy muscles and getting them ready for the day. Our "On the Bed" exercises will give you a feeling of energy and enthusiasm that ten cups of coffee can't provide. And the bed is a great place for stomach and leg work; after you've spent a few minutes revving up your whole body, take a few more and strengthen that tummy.

Think your morning shower or bath is only for washing the cobwebs out of your ears? Think again. "In the Tub" exercises can be done while soaking in a tub, showering, or toweling off. The bathtub is an ideal environment for exercise: warm water, like warm-ups, helps ready your muscles for a workout, making them 20 percent more effective. And the resistance of the water makes even the smallest movements count. Finish up with a tingling, stimulating rubdown using our toweling exercises.

At some point during the day, you probably wait in a line—a national pastime. At the bank and the post office, outside of movie theaters or in front of ticket windows —there are lines everywhere. Use these often irritating times to pick up your spirits and improve your fitness with our "Waiting in Line" exercises. They can be done so surreptitiously that no one will know why you're the only cheerful person in the queue. We've paid particular attention to the legs and feet, the areas most affected by standing for long periods of time; there are also some posture exercises that will help prevent backache and enable you to maintain your proud, upright stance.

Robert Kennedy used to drop to the floor of his office regularly and do thirty push-ups. Your own office might not lend itself to such a strenuous workout, but it's a great place for "At the Office" exercises. They can be done at your desk, at file cabinets, at the water cooler, even at the copier. Try some before that tricky sales meeting; they'll boost your energy and your spirits. They also help relieve tension, stress, stiff necks, upper and lower back spasms, cramps in your legs, and tension headaches —the adjuncts of a busy work day. You'll be more relaxed when you use these routines.

Is housework usually the least appealing task on your list? You'll breeze through it with our "Doing Housework" exercises. Developed while actually doing housework, these movements work while you sweep, mop, vacuum, wash dishes, do laundry, or even reach up into a kitchen cabinet or bedroom closet. Your normal movements are the foundations of these exercises; jobs that normally seem monotonous will become pleasurable little routines when you employ them.

Watching the evening news after a long day? Here's where you can really get down to it. Our "Watching TV" exercises are fairly strenuous, designed to work on your entire body. The slightly more complicated routines can neatly fit into your TV area, and will help you get through those dangerous commercial breaks without heading for the refrigerator. (Don't limit these exercises to evening viewing; they can be a great pick-me-up during morning news shows, too.)

Ready for bed? Discover something wonderful about our "On the Bed" exercises. Not only did they invigorate you in the morning—they can relax you at night. You'll sleep better if you repeat some of these stretches before you turn out the lights.

Heading for a vacation or a business trip? We've all experienced that dull, achy, "traveled out" feeling after long plane rides. The section "On a Train or Plane" can tell you how to exercise while you're seated in any confined space (you can use it when you're commuting, or sitting in a movie theater, or even waiting for the dentist—they'll calm you down). When you exercise in transit, you'll reach your destination feeling fresh as a daisy.

The exercises in this book contain both isometric and isotonic movements. (Isometric refers to the contraction and relaxation of muscles; they make up the more subtle exercises. Isotonics are movements in space.) We've also included a section called "Absolutely Anywhere" with routines that can fit in all those tight places. Be creative: don't limit yourself to the locations we've suggested. Many of these exercises can be adapted to fit into all your daily activities. And they have been specially designed so that you can easily do them in any type of clothing.

Combined with some sort of aerobic movement (see pages 24 and 108 for two "invisible" suggestions), they will provide you with a complete workout. They will tone and firm your body, strengthen and streamline your muscles, stimulate your circulation, and relieve stress and tension. You really can exercise anywhere—and in no time at all, you'll feel and look terrific.

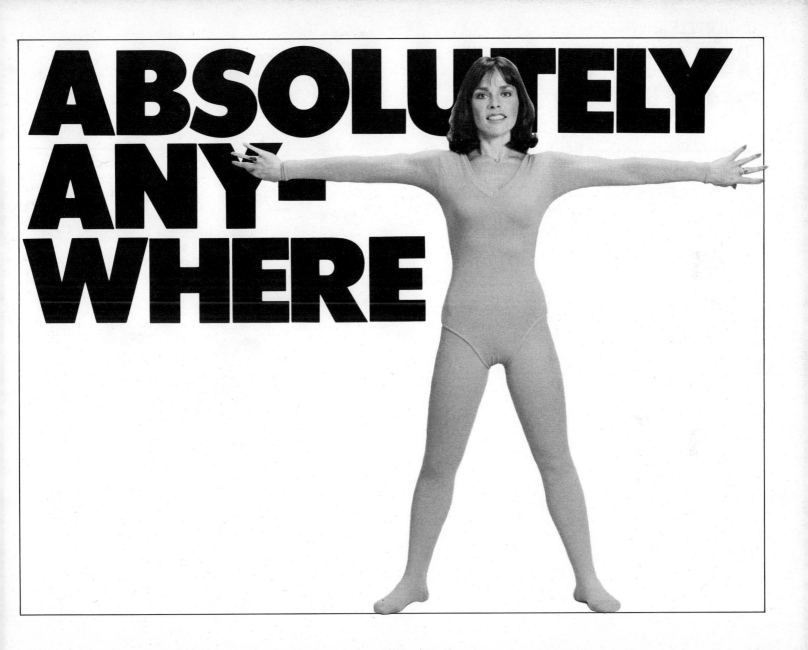

HEAD ROLLS

One of the all-time great exercises to relieve tension in the upper back, shoulders, and neck regions. Do it as often as you can—whether in part or all six steps. Turning to the left and right is excellent for keeping the jaw line smooth and well toned.

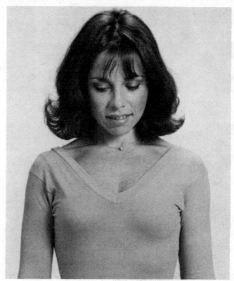

1

Stand (or sit) with a straight back, your legs slightly apart and your arms relaxed at your sides. Let your head drop forward.

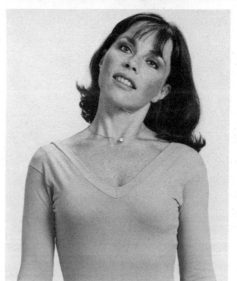

2

Rotate your head to the left, letting your chin pass over your left shoulder.

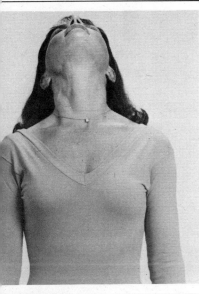

3

Continue to rotate your head to the back.

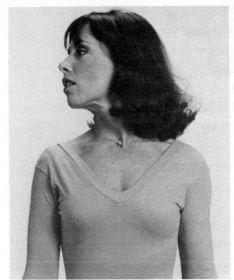

5

Keeping your torso still, turn your head as far to the right as you possibly can. Hold for 3 seconds.

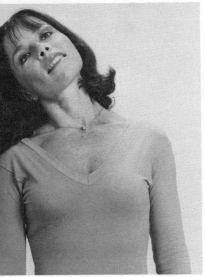

4

Rotate your head over your right shoulder and return to your original position. Repeat the rotation in the opposite direction.

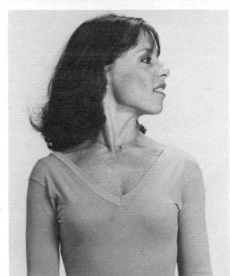

6

Turn your head as far to the left as you possibly can. Hold for 3 seconds. Repeat the sequence as often as you wish.

SHOULDER SHRUG

There's just no excuse for not doing this exercise, in cars, at desks, in the kitchen—even on the elevator. Tension from normal daily activities or stress builds in your upper back and shoulders. Release the tension with this simple workout.

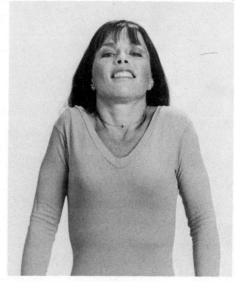

1
Stand (or sit) with a straight back, your feet slightly apart and your arms relaxed at your sides. Lift your shoulders as high as possible.

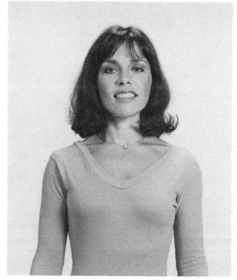

2
Lower your shoulders by pulling down with your hands.

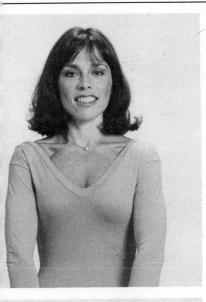

3

Without moving the rest of your body, begin a slow, rotating motion by rounding your shoulders forward.

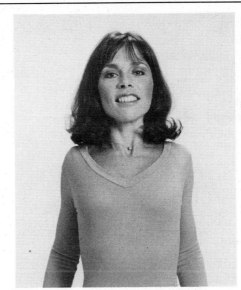

5

Stretch your shoulders back as far as possible, then lower them to a resting position. Repeat the sequence as often as you wish.

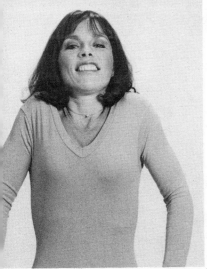

4

Lift your shoulders up toward your ears.

TORSO HUG WITH A TWIST

Even if you can't hold onto your waist in exactly this manner, you can still twist your torso to stretch your midriff. Keep your shoulders down and your stomach muscles tightened. Feel the gentle pull in your waist, midriff, and upper back.

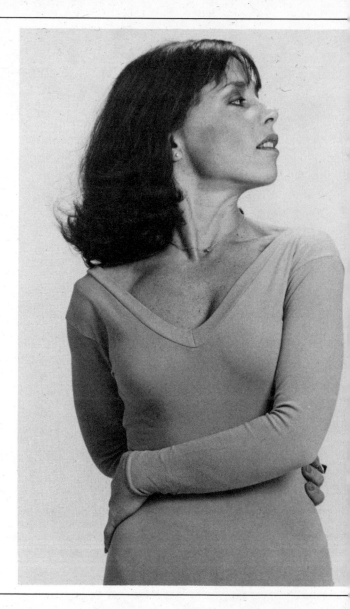

1

Stand straight with your legs together. Bend your left elbow and cross your left arm in front of you and hold onto your right side. Bend your right elbow and cross your right hand behind you and hold onto your left side. Keeping your torso still, turn your head as far to the left as you can.

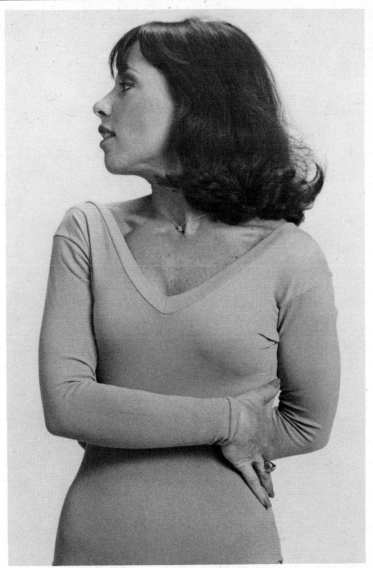

2

Change arms and turn your head as far to the right as you can. Repeat the sequence as often as you wish.

PUSH AND PULL

This exercise can be done anywhere, anytime—as long as your arms are free. It strengthens your pectoral muscles at the same time as it tones your upper arms.

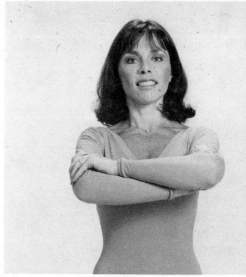

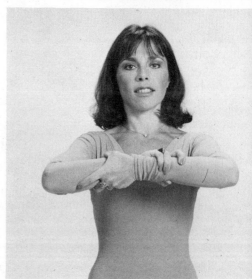

1

Stand straight
with your legs
slightly apart.
Cross your arms
in front of you at
shoulder level and
hold onto your
upper arms. Push
your hands against
your upper arms
and release 6
times.

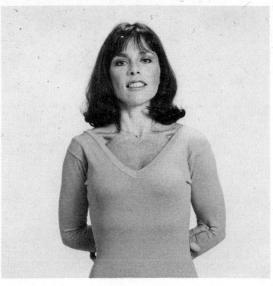

2

Keeping your arms
crossed in front of
you, hold onto your
wrists. Pull and
release 6 times.

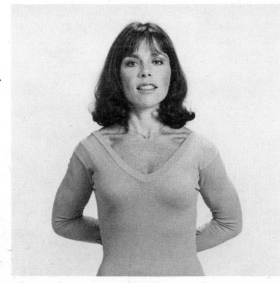

3

Cross your arms
behind you and
hold onto your
forearms. Push
and release 6
times.

4

With your arms
still crossed behind
you, hold onto your
wrists. Pull and
release 6 times.
Repeat the
sequence as often
as you wish.

SQUEEZE, STRETCH, AND TWIST

This hand-and-arm exercise relieves tension in your arms, back, and shoulders, as it tones and tightens your upper arms. You can work one arm at a time, if you're in cramped quarters—or holding onto a phone, shopping bag, or book.

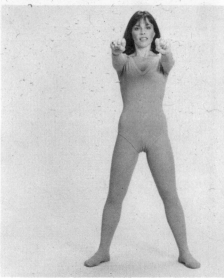

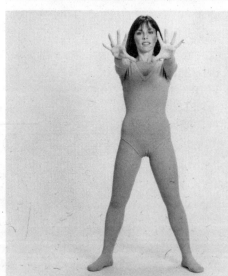

1

Stand (or sit) with a straight back, your feet about 18 inches apart and your arms extended in front at shoulder level. Make your hands into fists and squeeze for 3 seconds.

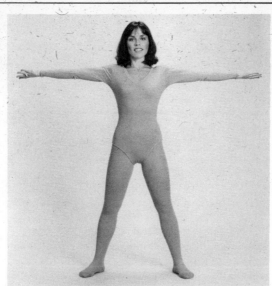

3

Stretch your arms out to the side at shoulder level. Turn the palms of your hands up, then back as far as possible, keeping your arms straight.

2

Open your fists and stretch your fingers as far apart as you can. Hold for 3 seconds.

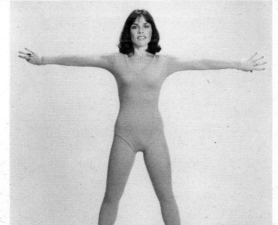

4

Turn your palms down, then back and up, so they face the ceiling. Repeat the sequence 6 times.

WALKING IN PLACE

Poor circulation, sore feet, stiff legs, and boredom are companions when waiting on line. Relieve all symptoms with this simple exercise. Keep your stomach muscles tightened and be sure to press down with the ball of your foot.

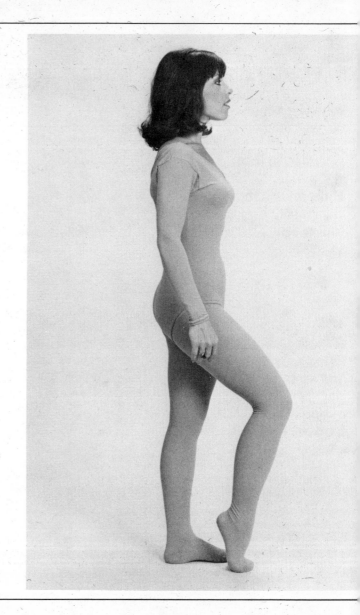

1

Stand with your legs straight, feet together, and arms relaxed at your sides. Raise your right heel, leaving the ball of your right foot on the floor.

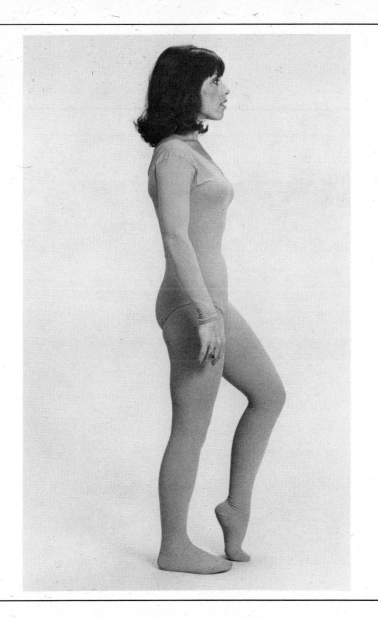

2

With a slow, steady motion, lower your right heel and lift your left heel off the floor. Raise and lower your heels in alternation whenever you wish.

TOE CURLS

Don't let standing in line waste your time. You're there for the duration, so use it to your advantage! Stretching and flexing your feet while standing—or while sitting, for that matter—stimulates circulation, soothes tired feet, and gives the calves a miniature workout.

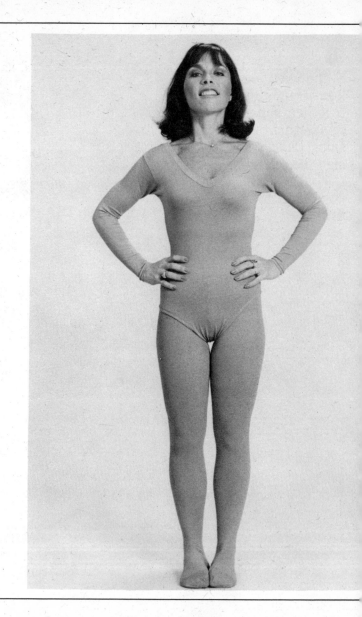

1

Stand with your
legs straight, feet
together, and arms
on your hips or
relaxed at your
sides. Curl your
toes under and
press your insteps
out, so your weight
rests on the
outsides of your
feet. Hold for 3
seconds.

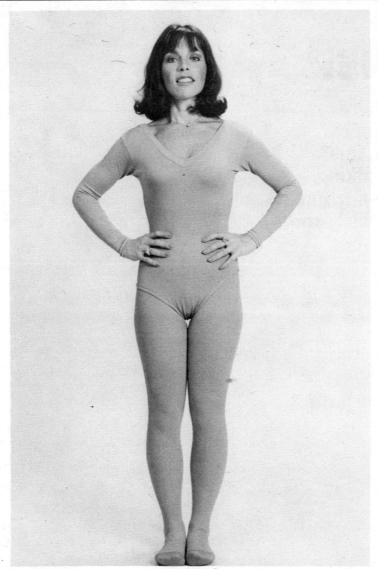

2

Flatten your feet
and flex your toes,
so they lift off the
floor. Hold for 3
seconds. Repeat
the sequence as
often as you wish.

THE TIGHTENER

No one will know you're firming and toning your buttocks but you. Do this exercise standing, walking, sitting, lying down—anytime, anywhere. Do it regularly and see your buttocks change shape.

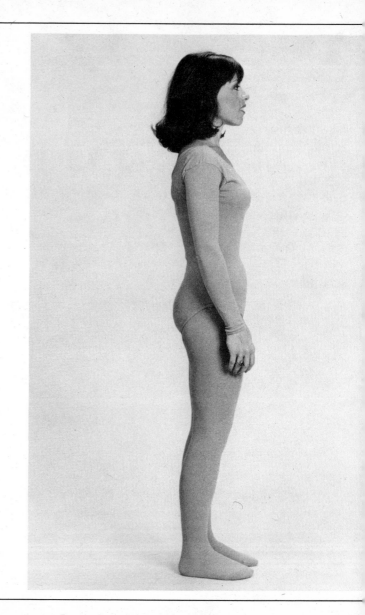

1

Stand straight
with your feet
slightly apart and
your arms relaxed
at your sides.

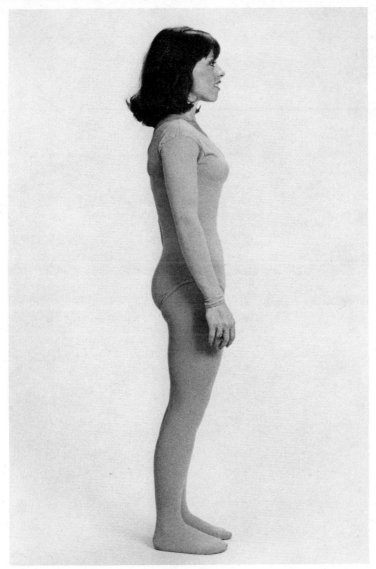

2

Pull in your
stomach and
tighten the
muscles in your
buttocks. Hold
this position for
5 seconds. Repeat
the sequence as
often as you wish.

ARCH AND FLATTEN, STANDING

Strong lower back muscles mean strong stomach muscles, and it is important to exercise both as often as you can. Make this simple workout a daily routine. It can be done in a chair or when standing, or lying down—as shown in the following exercise.

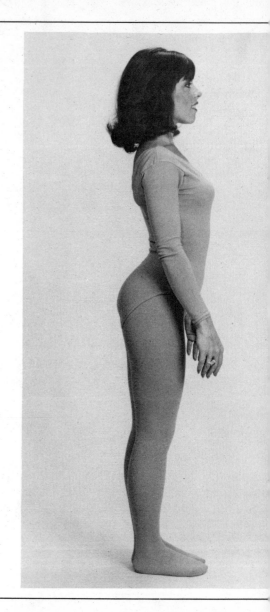

1

Stand straight
with your feet
together and your
arms relaxed at
your sides. Arch
your lower back
and stick out your
buttocks. Hold for
3 seconds.

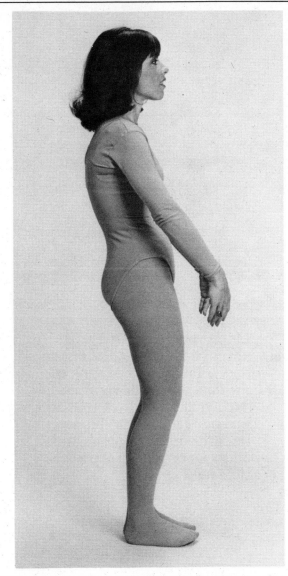

2

Slowly tuck your
buttocks under,
pushing your
pelvis forward and
upward. Keep your
stomach muscles
tightened. Hold for
3 seconds. Repeat
the sequence as
often as you wish.

ARCH AND FLATTEN, LYING DOWN

A variety of the standing Arch and Flatten to be done on your back. Do it often but never on the bed—only on the floor or a hard surface. It is excellent for relieving pain in the lower back and for relaxing tired or sore back muscles.

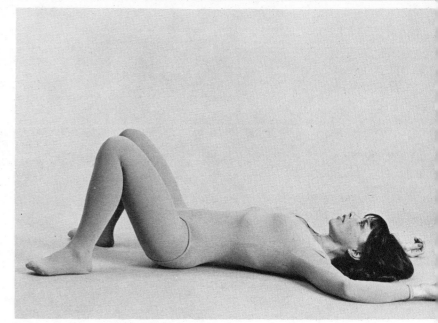

1 Lie on your back with your knees bent and feet flat on the floor. Place your forearms on the floor alongside your head. Arch your lower back so that it is about 2 inches off the floor. Be sure your upper back and buttocks remain on the floor. Hold for 3 seconds.

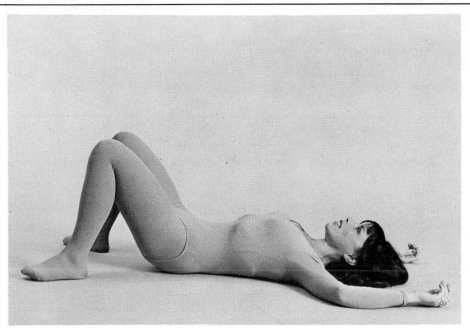

2 Tuck your pelvis under so that your lower back is pressed flat against the floor. Hold for 3 seconds and release. Repeat sequence as often as you wish.

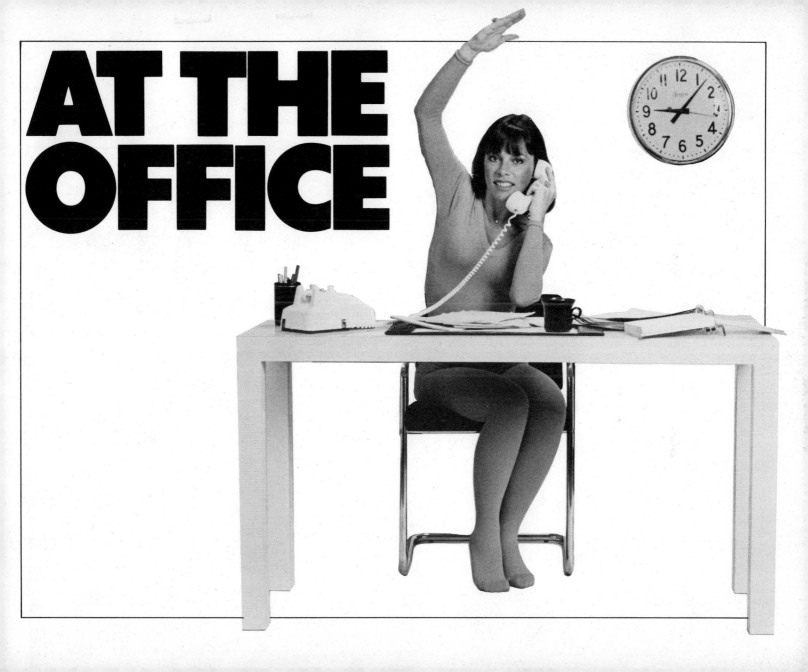

HEAD PRESS

Avoid a headache! This simple exercise releases building tension and renews energy before entering a sales meeting, balancing your checkbook, or dealing with junior. At any time at all. Be sure your head does the pressing, and not your hands.

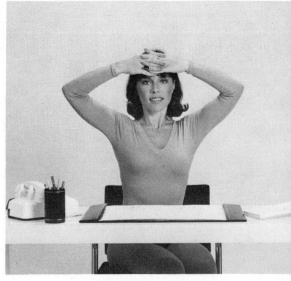

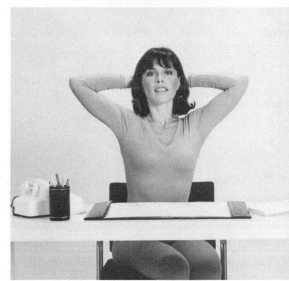

1

While sitting at the desk, lace your fingers and place your hands on your forehead. Without moving your hands, press your forehead against them for 3 seconds.

2

Keeping your fingers laced, place your hands behind your head. Press your head against your hands for 3 seconds.

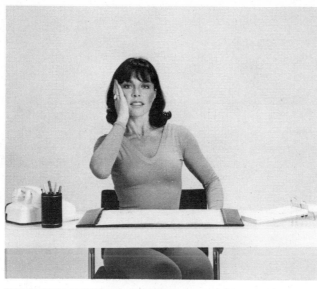

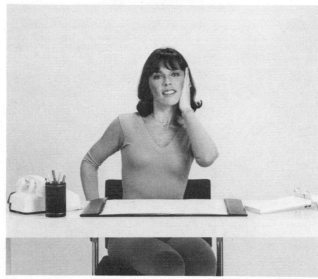

3

Place the palm of your right hand against your right cheek. Do not rest your elbow on the desk. Press your cheek against your palm for 3 seconds.

4

In the same manner, place your left palm on your left cheek and press for 3 seconds. Repeat the sequence 4 times.

TEN FINGER EXERCISE

Not even your fingers are immune from tension and stiffness. This exercise will relieve cramps and kinks in your hands and fingers, as well as give your pectoral muscles a miniature workout.

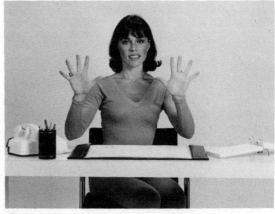

1 Sit (or stand) with your elbows bent and palms facing forward. Stretch your fingers and hold for 3 seconds.

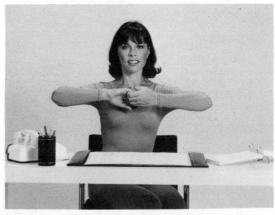

4 Now hook your fingers and pull with your arms as hard as you can for 3 seconds.

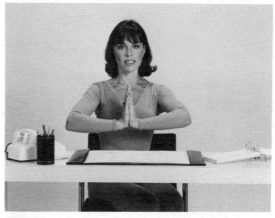

2 Make your hands into fists, and squeeze for 3 seconds.

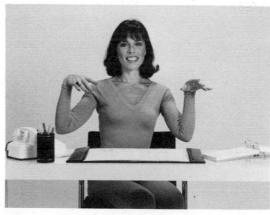

3 Open your hands and place your palms together in front of your chest, and press for 3 seconds.

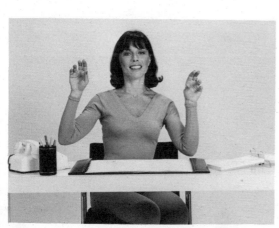

5 Return your hands to the original position of bent elbows. Wiggle your fingers for 3 seconds.

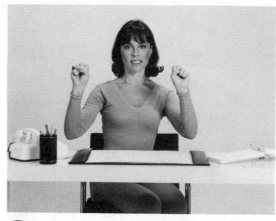

6 Shake your hands at the wrist for 3 seconds. Repeat the sequence 4 times.

THE BACK SCRATCH

Perfect for abating frustration when you are put on hold—or at the other end of an interminable conversation. This arm and shoulder exercise is especially good for posture. Steps 5 through 7 can be done separately and are effective in relieving tension in the upper back area.

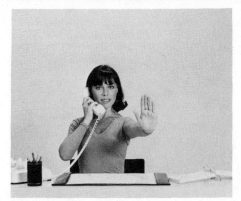

1 With the telephone in your right hand, stretch your left arm in front at shoulder level and flex your wrist.

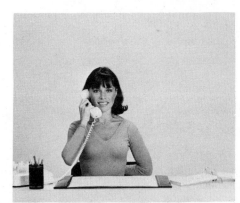

5 Bend your elbow and bring your hand behind your back, reaching as high as you can. Hold for 3 seconds.

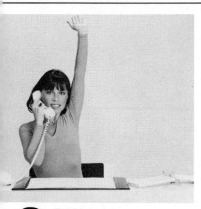

2 Raise your arm over head, pushing the heel of your palm to the ceiling.

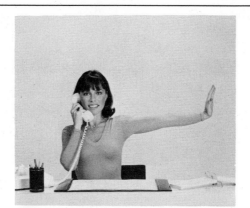

3 Lower your straight arm out to the side at shoulder level, continuing to push from the heel of your palm.

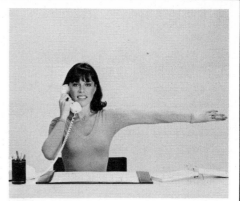

4 Keeping your arm stretched to the side, turn the palm back and then up so that the palm faces the ceiling.

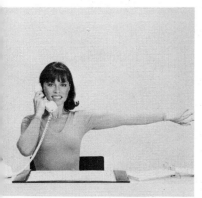

6 Bring your arm out to the side, turn your palm up and then back.

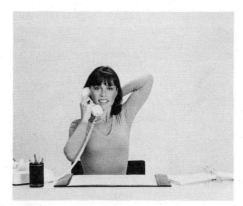

7 Bend and raise your elbow, lowering your hand. Hold for 3 seconds. Repeat with other arm.

LEG SWING

This easy swing is a gentle workout for your legs, while working at your desk or table. For best results, keep your toes pointed and hold your legs extended as long as you can.

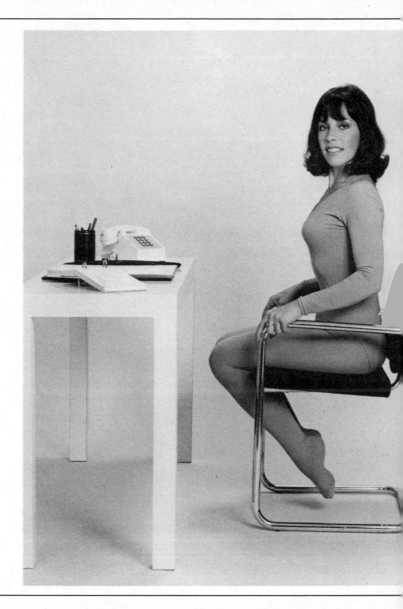

1

Sit with your back slightly away from the chair, with arms relaxed, or holding onto the chair or edge of the desk. With your feet pointed, press your calves as hard as you comfortably can against the bottom of the chair. Feel the pull in your upper thighs. Hold for 3 seconds.

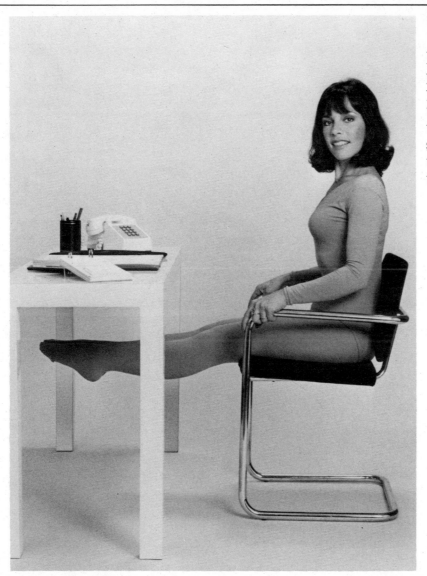

2

Keeping your feet pointed, straighten your legs so that they are parallel to the floor. Hold for 3 seconds. Repeat the sequence 8 times.

HIP LIFT

A good workout to keep those thighs from spreading—in any job or situation that requires sitting for long periods of time. Pulling your knee in to your chest also helps strengthen the lower back muscles.

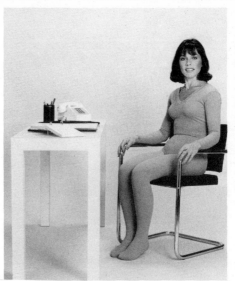

1

Sit in a chair with your back straight, legs together, and arms relaxed. If your chair has armrests, lightly hold onto them, or onto the edge of the desk.

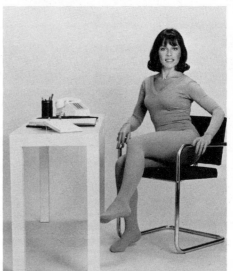

2

Keeping your left leg bent, lift your left hip off the chair. Your weight will be on your right thigh. Raise and lower your left hip 4 times.

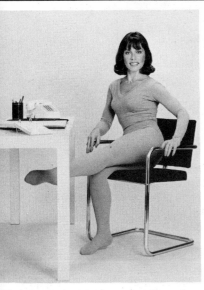

3

Now straighten your left leg and point your foot. In this position, raise and lower your left hip 4 times.

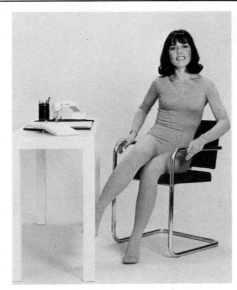

5

Change legs and repeat the sequence.

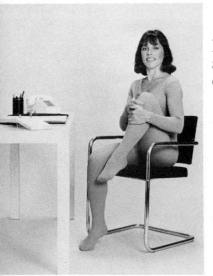

4

Lift your left knee and hug it to your chest for 3 seconds.

OFFICE PUSH-UP

Instead of taking a five-minute coffee break, relax with this exercise. It will relieve tension in the upper and lower back—and, if you keep your stomach muscles tightened, will help keep your stomach firm.

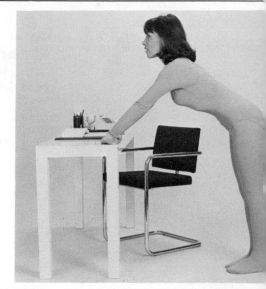

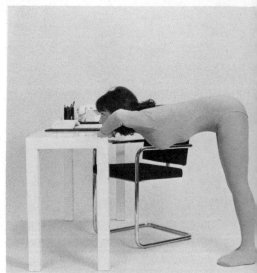

1

Standing with your legs together and about 3 feet from the desk, place your palms flat on the desk, fingertips touching. Be sure your arms and back are straight and your stomach muscles tightened.

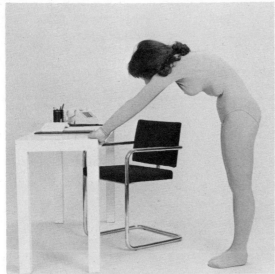

3

Slowly straighten your arms, lifting your torso and rounding your back. Hold for 3 seconds.

2

Slowly bend your elbows and bring your chin to the desk, so that your back is straight and parallel to the floor. Do not lift your heels off the floor. Hold for 3 seconds.

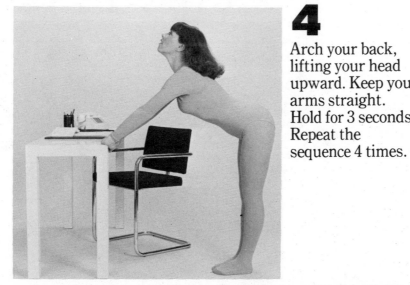

4

Arch your back, lifting your head upward. Keep your arms straight. Hold for 3 seconds. Repeat the sequence 4 times.

COPY ME

Standing at a copier is a perfect time to give your legs a workout. Be sure to keep your stomach muscles tightened. Try to lift your leg higher each time you do this exercise.

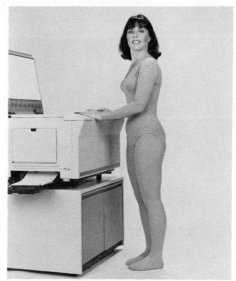

1

Stand with your legs straight, feet slightly apart, and arms relaxed at your sides or resting on the copier.

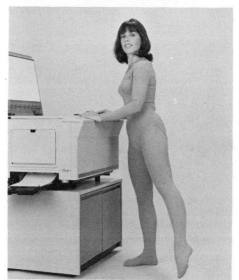

2

Keeping your left leg straight, with your foot pointed, lift it to the side 4 times . . .

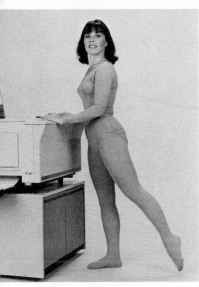

3

...then to the back
4 times.

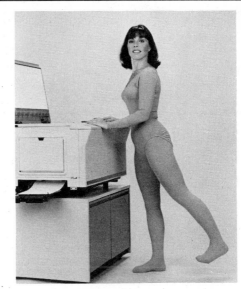

5

...and to the back
4 times. Repeat the
sequence 4 times
with each leg.

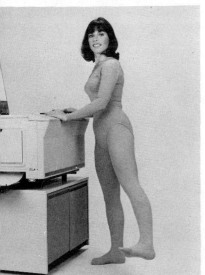

4

Flex your left foot
and, in the same
manner, lift it to
the side 4 times...

JOGGER'S STRETCH

You don't have to jog to get cramps in your legs! Leg muscles shorten and become tight in the calves and behind the knees from high heels and excessive sitting. Use your time at the copier to stretch out the muscles in the backs of your legs. Be sure to keep the foot of your straight leg flat on the floor, for maximum tendon and muscle stretch.

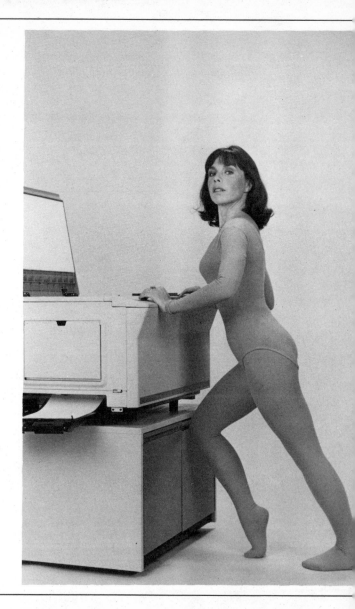

1

Stand about 2 feet from the copier, with right leg forward. Raise your right heel, leaving only the ball of your right foot on the floor. Keep your body and left leg straight and your stomach muscles tightened.

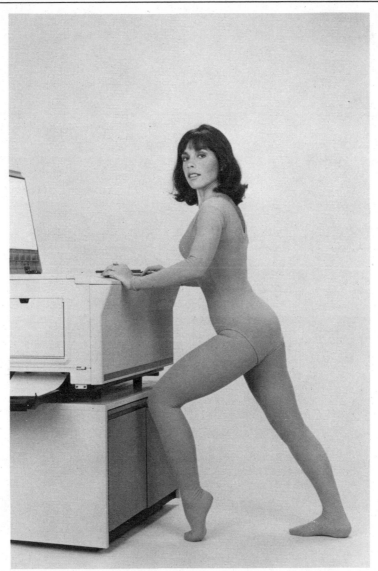

2

With a slow steady motion, lower your right heel, reverse legs, and lift your left heel off the floor. Raise and lower your heels, in alternation, at least 8 times—or until the job is finished.

FILE AWAY

This exercise is difficult unless you have a filing cabinet (or dresser or cupboard drawer) to hold onto—and the time to spend stretching your legs while you work. It is excellent, however, for increasing the strength and flexibility of your legs.

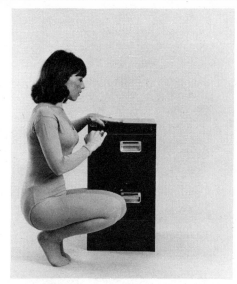

1

Stand with your legs straight and together about 12 inches from the filing cabinet. Holding onto the cabinet, bend your knees, so that your heels lift off the floor and your buttocks rest on your ankles.

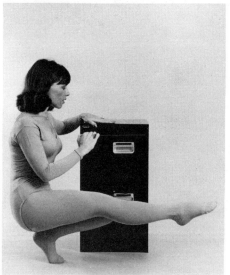

2

Keeping your back straight, extend your right leg with foot pointed. Your weight should be on the ball of your left foot.

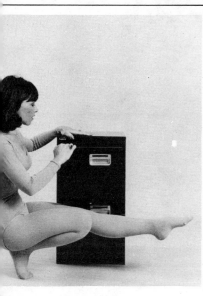

3

Reverse legs and
extend your left
leg.

4

Extend your right
leg again, but with
a flexed foot ...

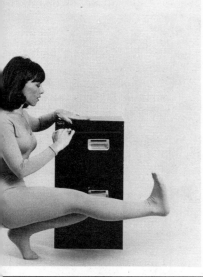

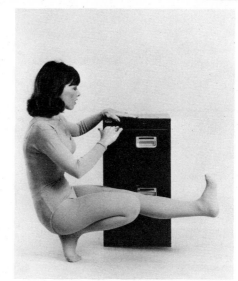

5

...and then your
left leg with foot
flexed. Repeat the
sequence, if you
can.

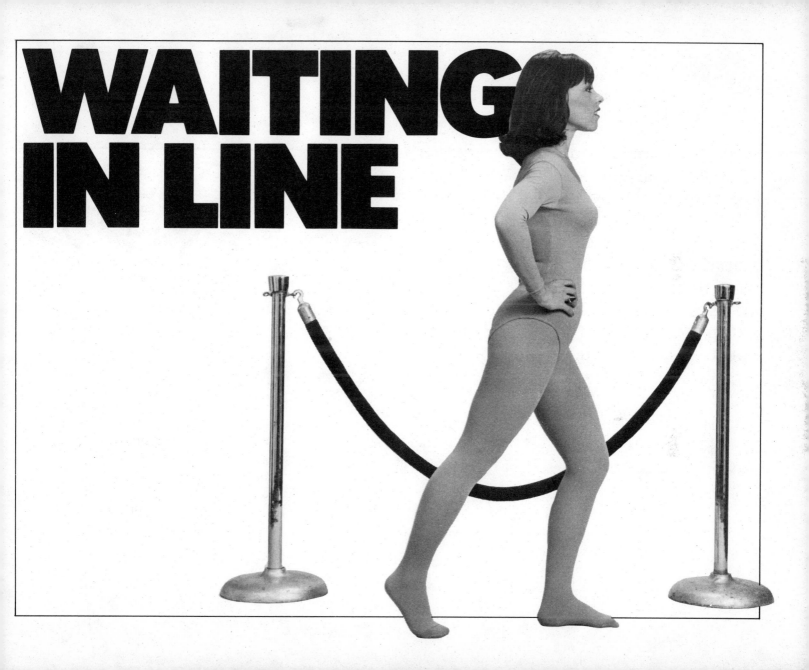

ON GUARD

Don't rock back and forth in line aimlessly. Make those movements and your idle time work for you. This exercise is excellent for circulation and for toning and firming thigh and calf muscles. For added benefits, keep your stomach and buttocks tightened.

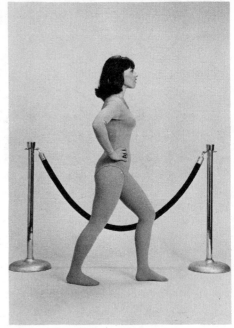

1 Stand with your left foot about 18 inches in front of your right leg. Your left knee should be slightly bent, your back straight, and your hands on your waist or relaxed at your sides.

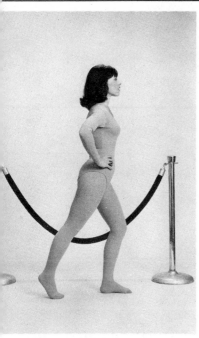

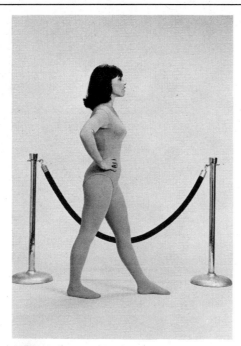

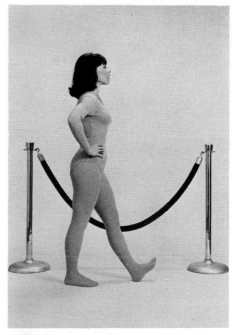

2 Lift your right heel off the floor and shift your weight onto your left foot. Keep your left knee bent. Hold for 3 seconds.

3 Lower your right heel and straighten your left knee.

4 Shifting your weight to your left leg lift your right foot, keeping the heel on the floor. Hold for 3 seconds. Be sure to stretch the back of your right leg. Repeat the sequence 6 times with each leg.

UP AND DOWN

Make the most of those minutes standing in line. This easy knee bend and slow leg stretch on toe works the entire leg and your stomach muscles, if you keep them tightened. Excellent for posture and balance, too.

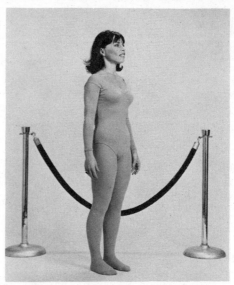

1
Stand straight with your feet slightly apart. Keep your shoulders down and your arms relaxed at your sides.

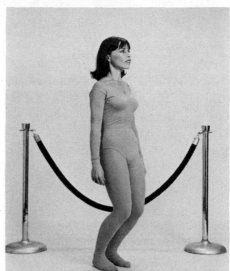

2
Bend your knees and lower your torso about 12 inches. Be sure to keep your heels flat on the floor and your back straight. Hold for 3 seconds.

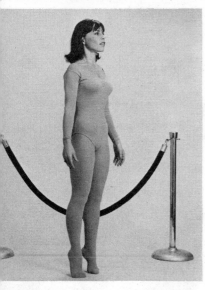

3

Rise slowly onto the balls of your feet. Hold for 3 seconds, then lower your heels.

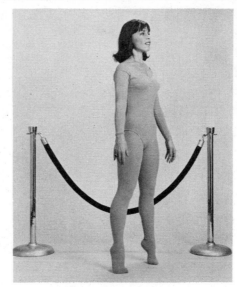

5

Rise onto the balls of your feet and hold for 3 seconds. Repeat the sequence 6 times.

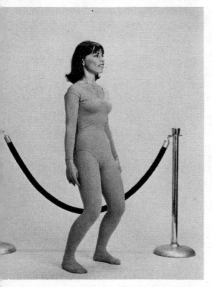

4

Place your feet about 18 inches apart. Bend your knees and lower your torso about 12 inches, keeping your stomach and buttocks muscles tightened. Hold for 3 seconds.

ATTENTION-GETTER

Similar to a knee bend and stretch, this exercise not only enhances balance and posture, but gives your ankles and arms a workout. Be careful not to nudge the person in front or in back.

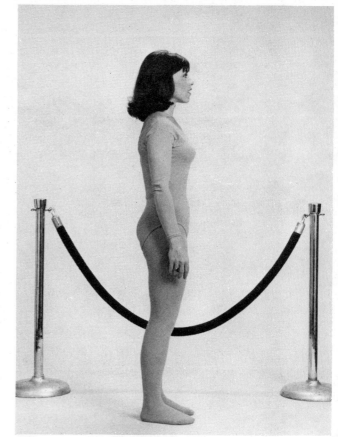

1 Stand straight with your feet slightly apart and your arms at your sides.

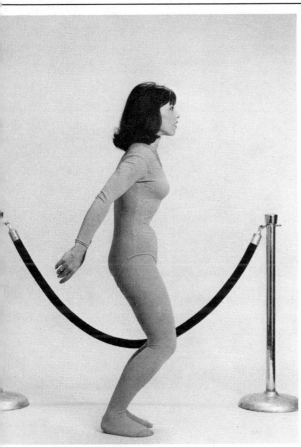

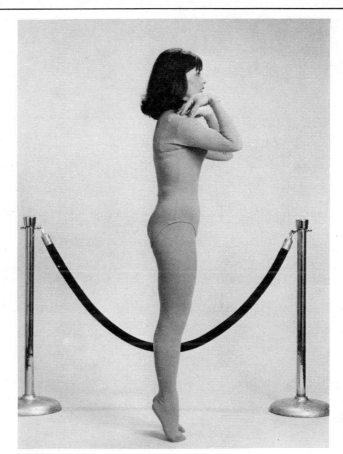

2 Slightly bend your knees and swing your arms straight in back of you. Keep your heels on the floor.

3 In one continuous motion, straighten your legs and go up on your toes, as you swing your arms forward and up, so that your fingertips rest on your shoulders. Repeat the sequence 6 times.

FLEX, BEND, AND PULL

Everyone wants a slim and trim waist, and this easy exercise can help. The stretch tightens the midriff and the pull tones the waist.

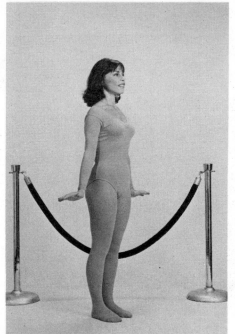

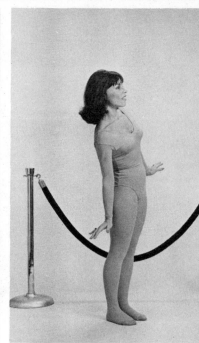

1 Stand straight with your feet slightly apart. Your arms should be at your sides with your wrists flexed. Without moving your body, push down with the heels of your palms for 3 seconds.

2 Keeping your wrists flexed, bend from the waist as far to the right as you can. Continue to push with the heels of your palms. Do not lean forward.

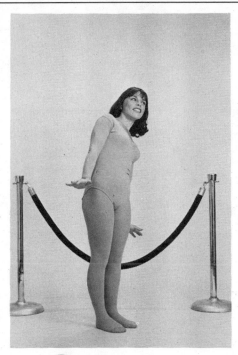

3 In the same manner, bend to the left.

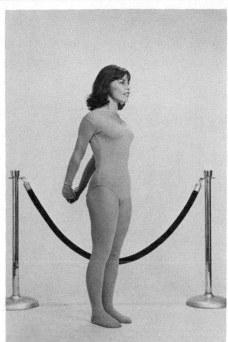

4 Clasp your hands tightly behind your buttocks and pull down from your shoulders. Your upper back will arch slightly.

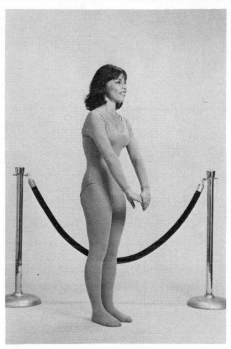

5 Clasp your hands in front of you and pull down from your shoulders. Your shoulders will be rounded slightly. Repeat the sequence 4 times.

TWIST AND TILT

People will think you are looking for someone, but actually you are giving your waist, midriff, and stomach muscles a mini-workout. Your arms can be relaxed at your sides, but your stomach and buttocks muscles must be tightened. Do not move your hips.

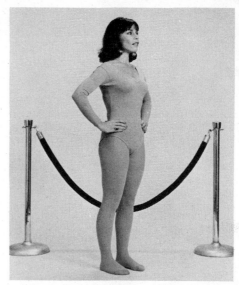

1
Stand straight with your feet slightly apart and your hands on your waist.

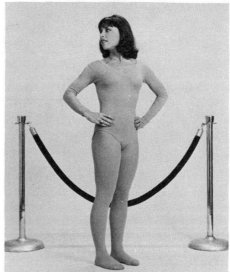

2
Twist your torso as far to the right as you can. Keep your hips and legs still.

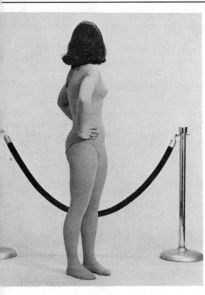

3

In the same manner, twist to the left.

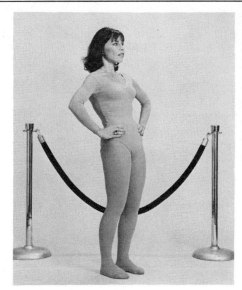

5

Keeping your buttocks tucked under, tilt backward. Do not arch your back. Repeat the sequence 4 times.

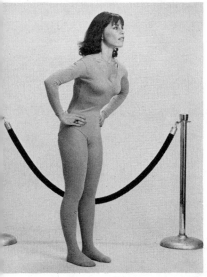

4

Tuck your buttocks under and tilt forward from the waist. Keep your back straight and your head up.

MIDRIFF SLIDE

While doing this relaxing but effective exercise, be sure to keep your stomach muscles tightened, your hips still, and your shoulders down. Enjoy the slow slide.

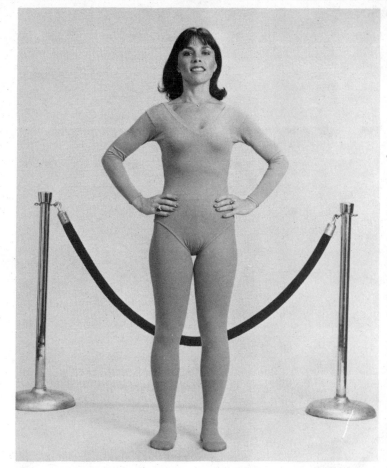

1 Stand straight with your feet slightly apart and your hands on your waist.

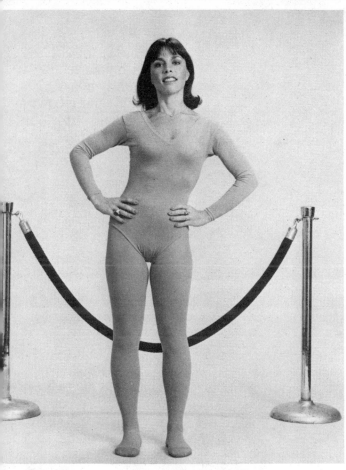

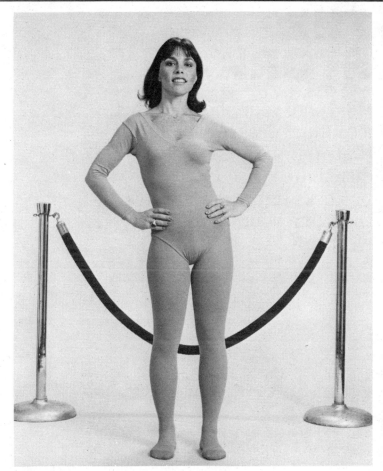

2 Without moving your hips, slide your torso as far to the left as you can. Keep your shoulders level.

3 Slide your torso to the right, again without moving your hips. Repeat the sequence as often as you wish.

THE STORK

Hold onto your shopping cart, a counter, desk, or chair, so that your weight is evenly distributed. Keep your buttocks tightened and give them and your thighs a real workout.

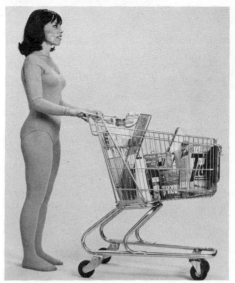

1

Stand straight with your feet slightly apart. Bend your elbows and hold onto your shopping cart handle.

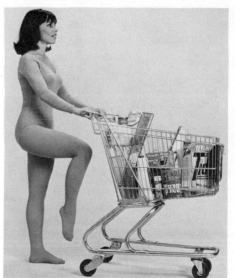

2

Bend your right knee and lift your leg, so it forms a right angle to the floor. Keep your foot pointed. Hold for 3 seconds.

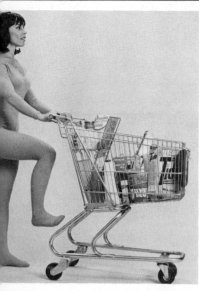

3

Keeping your right leg in this raised position, flex your right foot. Hold for 3 seconds.

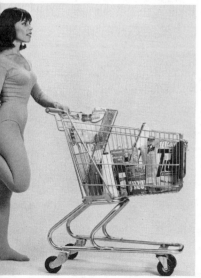

4

Clasp your right ankle with your right hand and bring your right heel as close to your buttocks as you can. Hold for 3 seconds.

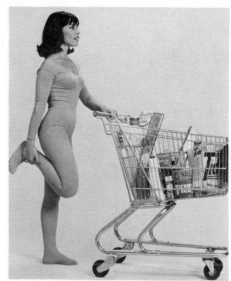

5

Flex your foot and hold for 3 seconds. Repeat the sequence 4 times with each leg.

CART STRETCH

An exercise no one will know you're doing! Stretch while loading or unloading a grocery cart or when you must reach for something a short distance away. Keep your stomach muscles tightened and your legs straight.

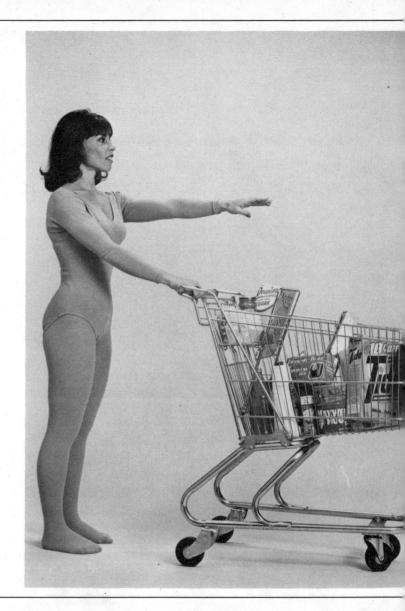

1

Stand straight
with your feet
slightly apart.
Keeping your arms
straight, hold onto
the cart with your
right hand and
extend your left
arm at shoulder
level.

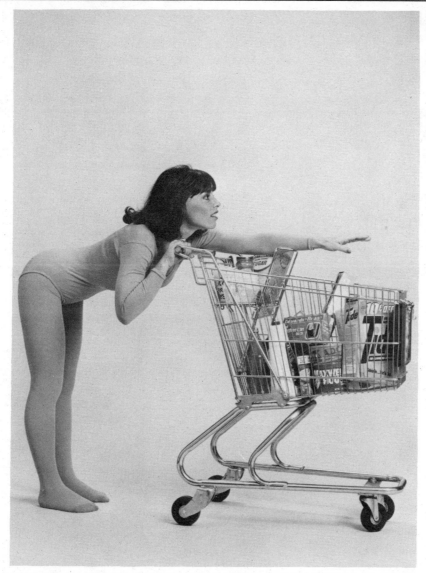

2

Bend at the hips
and reach forward
with your left
arm as far as you
comfortably can.
Your back should
be straight and
your right elbow
bent. Change arms
and extend your
right arm as far as
you can. Repeat
the sequence 6
times.

STRETCH AND BEND

Again, hold onto your shopping cart or a counter while you bend and stretch your legs. Be sure to keep your buttocks and back straight. For extra toning, try to hold the bent-knee position for as long as you can.

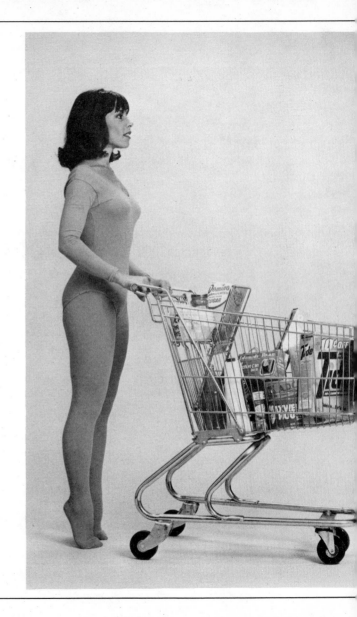

1

Stand straight
with your feet
slightly apart.
Bend your elbows
and hold onto your
shopping cart with
your hands. Raise
your heels off the
floor so that your
weight rests on the
balls of your feet.
Hold for 3 seconds.

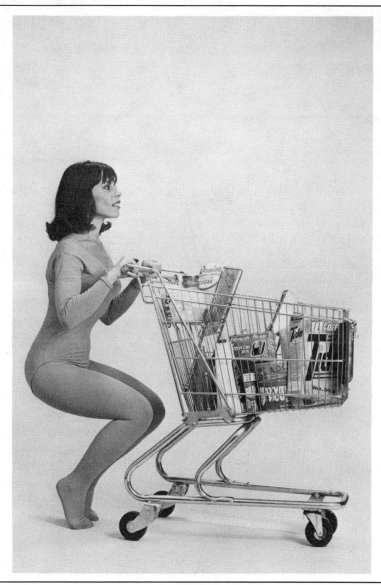

2

Holding onto the
shopping cart and
keeping your heels
off the floor, bend
your knees and
lower your torso,
so your thighs are
parallel to the
floor. Without
lowering your
heels to the floor,
repeat the
sequence 6 times.

ON A TRAIN OR PLANE

ELBOWS BACK

Excellent for relieving tension in the upper back, when sitting still for a long period of time. This exercise will also relax shoulder muscles after carrying heavy suitcases, shoulder bags, or packages. It can be done standing as well. Wherever, whenever, it is best to keep stomach muscles tightened.

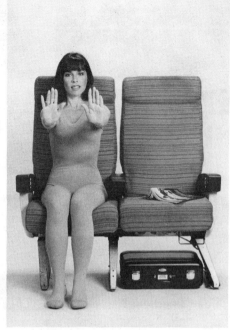

1 Sit in a chair with your back straight and your legs together. Stretch your arms in front of you at shoulder level, and flex your wrists. Push the heels of your palms forward, but do not move your shoulders or arms.

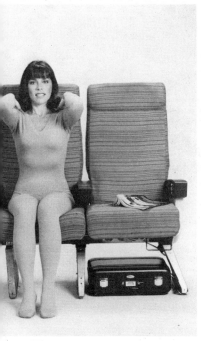

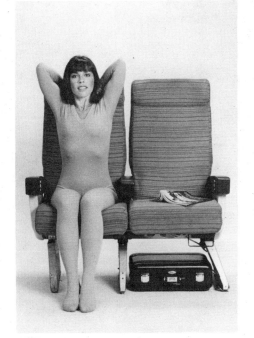

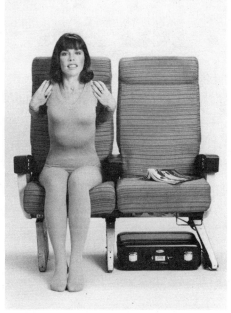

2 Bend your elbows and rest your fingertips on your shoulders.

3 Keeping your back straight and your head still, raise your elbows so they point upward. Hold for 3 seconds.

4 Bring your elbows down and back, keeping your arms as close to the torso as possible. Hold for 3 seconds. Repeat the sequence 8 times.

TWIST AND TURN

Talking to two people on either side of you at the same time might make you feel as if you are watching a championship tennis match. Use the opportunity to stretch your torso and work your midriff. It is important to keep your back straight and your stomach muscles tightened.

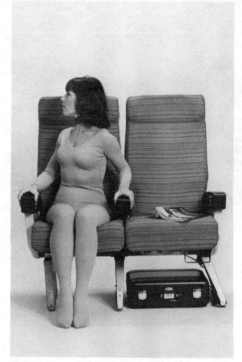

1 Sit in a chair with your legs together and your hands on the armrests. Keeping your back straight, twist your torso as far to the right as you can.

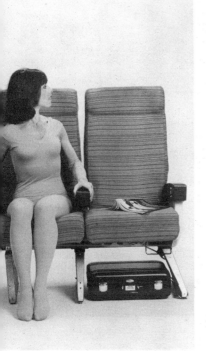

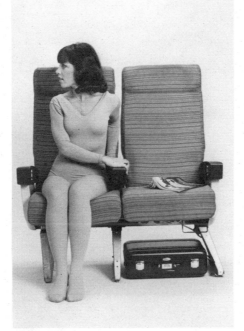

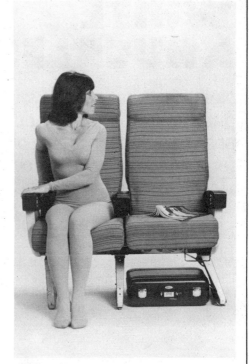

2 In the same manner, twist your torso to the left. Twist to the right and to the left 4 times.

3 Hold the left armrest with both hands. Twist your torso as far to the right as you can. Be sure your back is straight.

4 Hold the right armrest with both hands and twist your torso as far to the left as you can. Repeat steps 3 and 4 at least 4 times.

WHITE KNUCKLES

Neighbors may think you are practicing the crash landing position—or perhaps looking for something on the floor. However, you are really relieving tension in your hands, arms, and back. Lowering your head helps circulation.

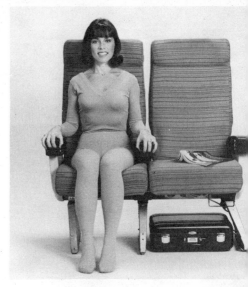

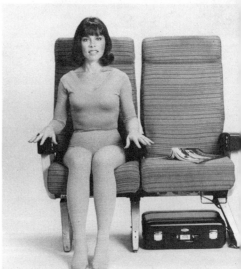

1

Sit in an armchair with your back straight and your stomach muscles tightened. Hold the ends of the chair arms and squeeze firmly.

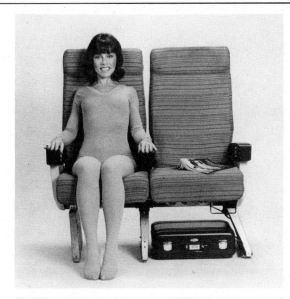

3

While pressing your lower back against the chair, arch your upper back and hold for 3 seconds.

2

Release your hands and stretch out your fingers. Squeeze and release 8 times.

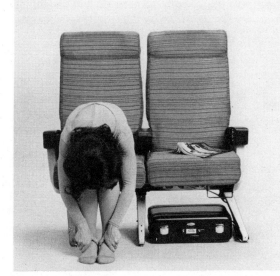

4

Bend at the waist and clasp your ankles with your hands. With a round back, pull your torso down to your thighs. Be sure your stomach muscles are tightened. Hold for 3 seconds. Repeat steps 3 and 4 at least 6 times.

STRETCH AND HUG

Stretching is essential for good body tone and can be done lying down, standing up, or sitting in a chair. This exercise is perfect for those times when you're glued to a chair for a long period. It helps you to "stretch out" the torso, arms, and legs, as well as to relax cramped muscles.

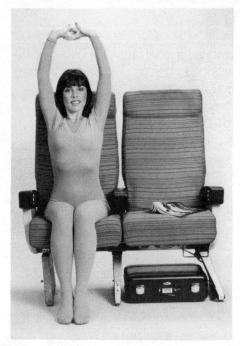

1 Sit in an armchair with your back straight. Lace fingers and stretch your arms over your head so that the palms face up. Hold the stretch for 3 seconds.

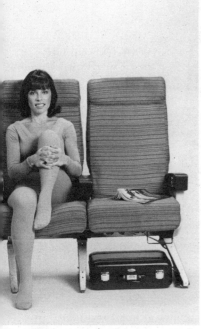

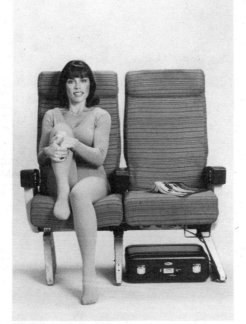

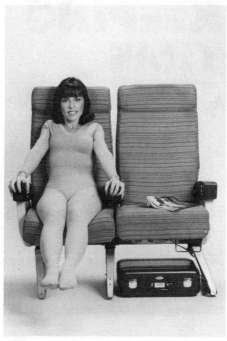

2 Bring your left knee to your chest and clasp your hands around it. Be sure to keep your back straight and your left foot pointed. Hug your knee to your chest for 3 seconds.

3 Lower your left leg as you bring your right knee to your chest and hug it to your chest for 3 seconds.

4 In one continuous movement, grip the chair arms and push against the back of the chair, straightening your arms and stretching your legs. Your feet should lift off the floor. Hold for 3 seconds and release. Repeat the sequence 4 times.

KEEPING TIME

Your leg muscles will know they are having a workout but your neighbor won't, as you do this exercise while reading a book, or watching a movie or television on the plane. "Keeping Time" will stimulate circulation throughout the leg and help keep ankles trim.

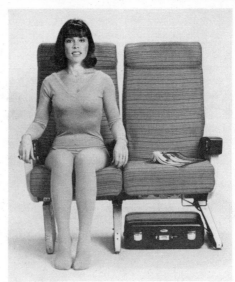

1

Sit in a chair with your toes on the floor and your heels slightly raised. Keep your back straight and your stomach muscles tightened.

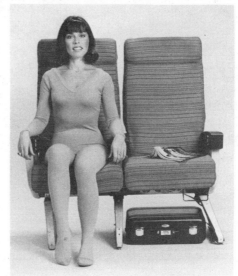

2

Slowly lower your left heel to the floor.

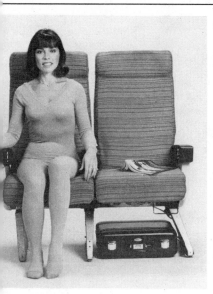

3

With a slow, steady motion, lower your right heel while you lift your left heel off the floor. Raise and lower your heels, alternating, 8 times, then place both feet on the floor.

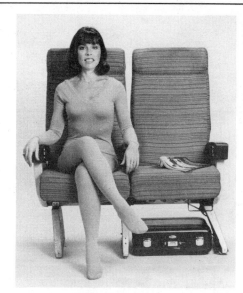

5

Point your right foot downward as far as possible. Flex and point your right foot 8 times.

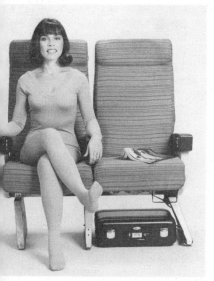

4

Cross your right leg over your left and flex your right foot.

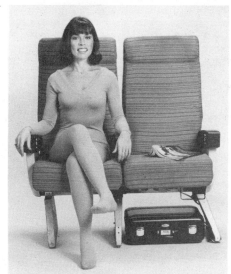

6

Rotate your right foot from the ankle in 4 clockwise circles, then in 4 counterclockwise circles. Reverse legs and repeat steps 4 through 7 with your left foot.

THE LONG STRETCH

When you feel you're going to jump out of your skin from sitting too long, slowly stretch out your entire body to relieve tension and cramped muscles. Try to form a perfectly straight line with your body.

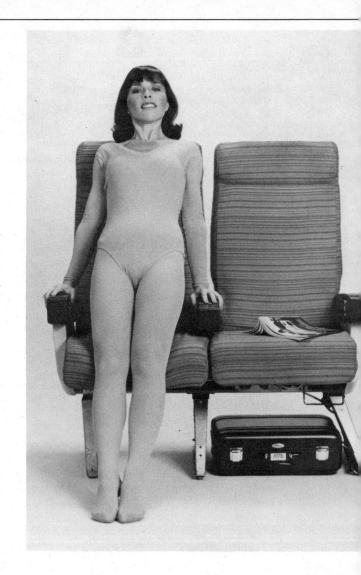

1

Begin in a sitting position, with your hands gripping the armrests, and your legs stretched out in front of you. Lift your torso off the chair and straighten your arms so your body forms a straight line. Do not bend your elbows or allow your head to fall back. Hold for 3 seconds.

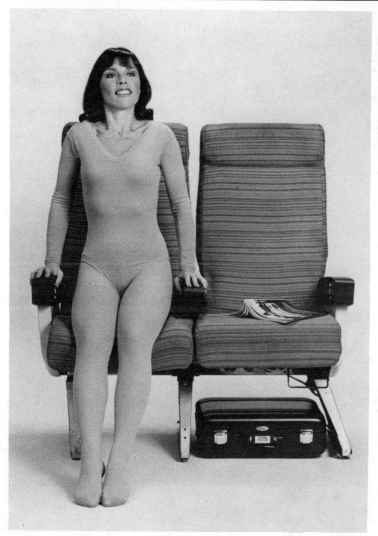

2

Bend your elbows and slowly lower your body, buttocks first, into a sitting position. Repeat the sequence 8 times.

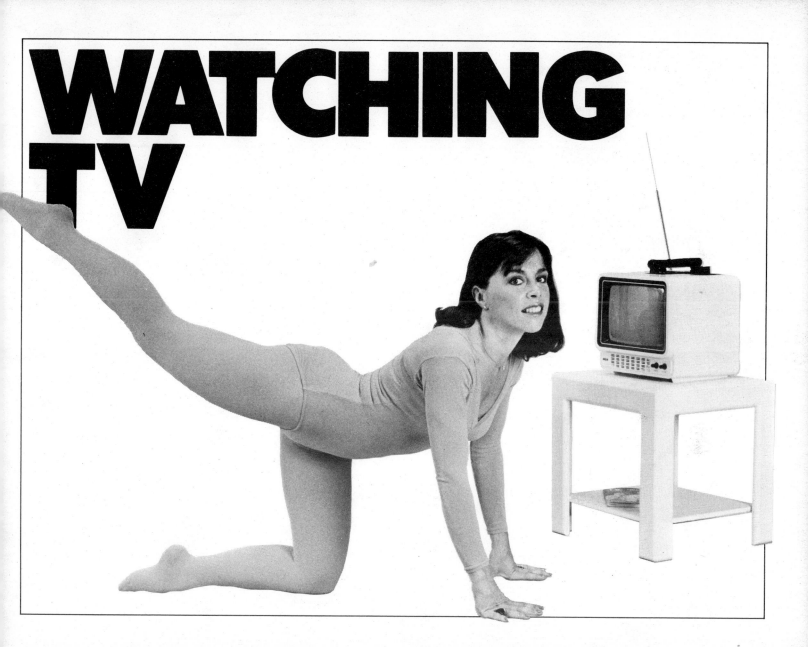

WATCHING TV

TV SIT-UP

Sit-ups are never much fun, but they are tolerable if done while watching your favorite television program and, if you like, bracing your feet under a stationary table, chair, or sofa. The sit-up is one of the best exercises for toning and firming stomach muscles.

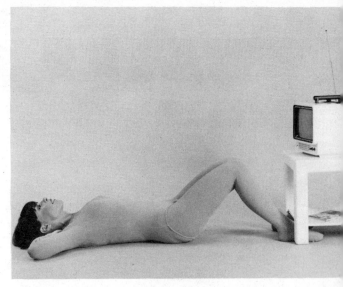

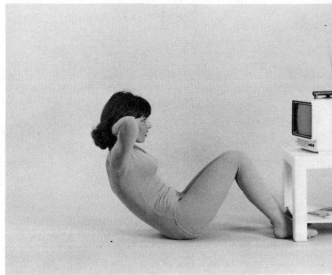

1

Lie flat on your back with knees bent and slightly apart. Your feet should be flat on the floor and, if necessary, anchored under a table or chair. Clasp your hands behind your neck.

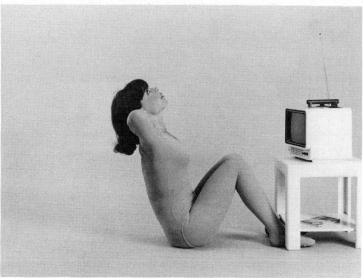

2

Tighten your stomach muscles and slowly bring your torso up into a sitting position, with your back rounded. Keep feet flat on the floor.

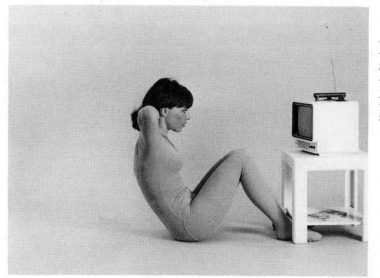

3

When you reach a sitting position, straighten your back, and lift your face to the ceiling.

4

Round your back and slowly lower your torso to the floor. Repeat the sequence 8 times.

BUTTOCKS WALK

Most people think this exercise is for the buttocks. Wrong! You are actually using and tightening your stomach muscles. Do it while watching television, or, as a few of my students do, while reading a book.

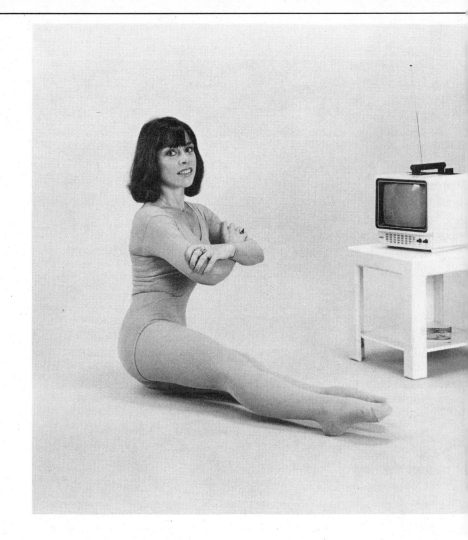

1

Sit on the floor with your legs and back straight and your feet pointed. Your arms should be extended at shoulder level and crossed in front of your chest. Keeping your legs straight, "walk" on your buttocks, by lifting your right hip and leg.

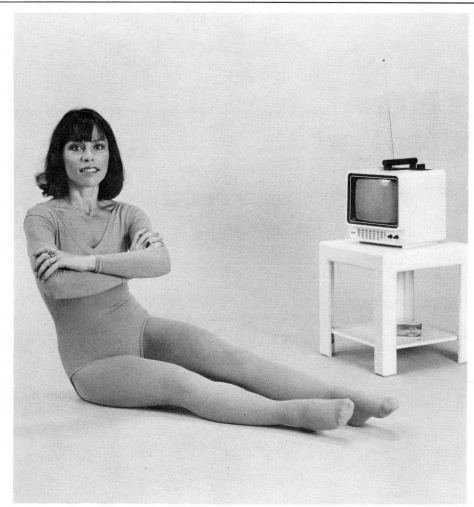

2

In the same manner, lift your left hip and leg. "Walk" as far forward as you can in one direction, and then "walk" backward to your original position.

SIT-UP CROSS-OVER AND STRETCH

Everyone knows you can flatten your stomach with sit-ups. In this exercise, you give your stomach a similar workout, as you tone and firm your midriff and upper arms.

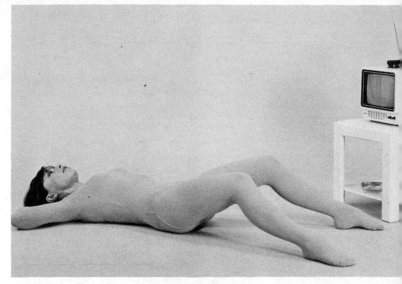

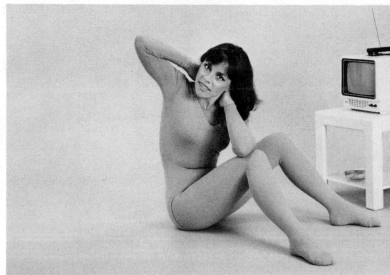

1

Lie on your back with your knees bent and feet flat on the floor. Your feet should be about 18 inches apart. Clasp your hands behind your neck.

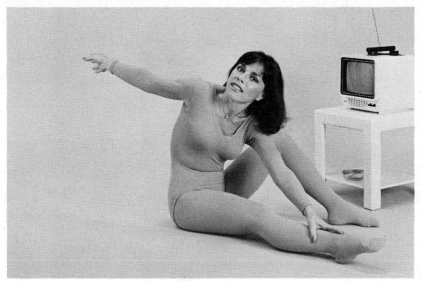

3

In one continuous motion, straighten your right leg and clasp the ankle with your left hand, as you reach directly back with your right arm.

2

With your hands clasped behind your neck and your feet flat on the floor, sit up and twist your torso, touching your left elbow to your right knee.

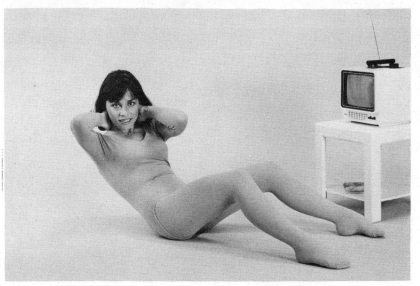

4

Return to the original position. Repeat the sequence 6 times, alternating sides.

BODY FOLDS

Exercise can be serious work —especially this one for your stomach muscles. You may not be able to repeat this exercise four times in the beginning, but stay with it until you can. The results are worth it!

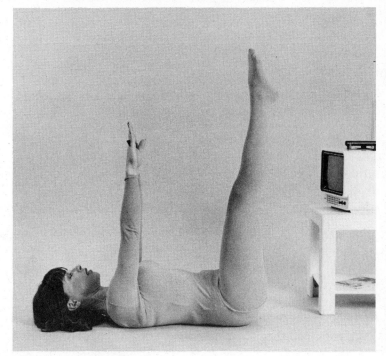

1 Lie flat on your back with your arms and legs stretched straight up in the air, so that your body forms a U. Your feet should be pointed.

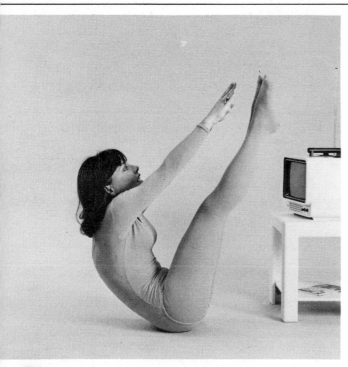

2 Keeping your stomach pulled in, lift your back and torso off the floor and reach for your feet, all in one movement.

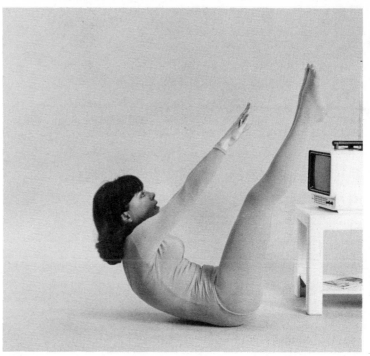

3 Relax to the original position, making sure to keep your arms and legs perpendicular to the floor. Repeat the sequence 4 times.

HIP ROLL

This hip roll exercises your thighs and stomach muscles. For best results, keep your legs off the floor and your stomach muscles tightened. Try to hold your position in Step 3 as long as you can.

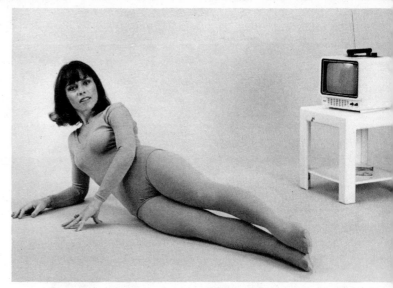

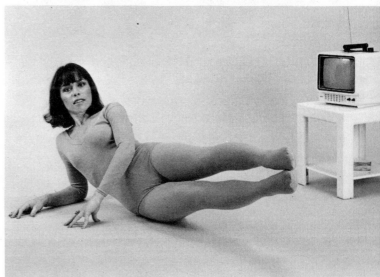

1

Lie on your right side with your torso propped up on your right elbow. Place your left arm in front of you with fingers on the floor. Your legs should be straight and feet pointed.

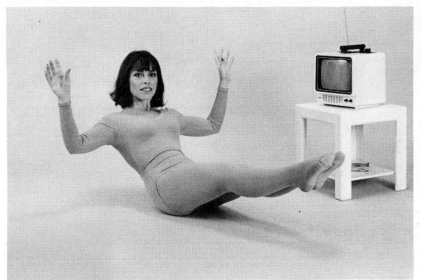

3

Without lowering your legs, roll onto your buttocks and lift your arms, so that your forearms are parallel to your head. Keep your stomach and buttocks muscles tightened and your legs off the floor. Hold.

2

Lift your legs about 12 inches from the floor. Stretch your legs and make them as long as possible.

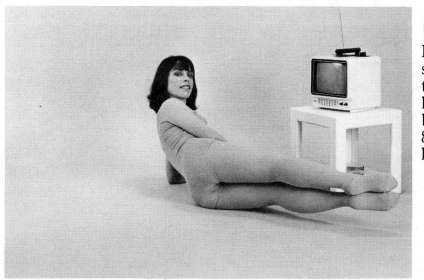

4

Roll onto your left side and prop your torso up on your left elbow. Roll back and forth 8 times without lowering your legs.

SWING BLADE TO KICK

This exercise may take a little more room than others, so be careful of the furniture and lamps. It is, however, excellent for toning and firming the legs and hips.

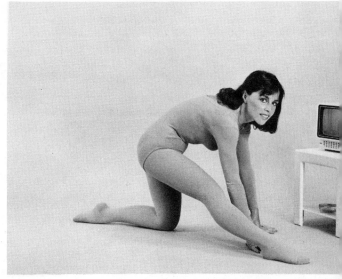

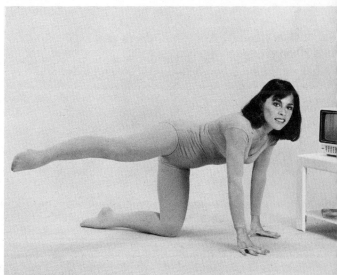

1

Beginning on your hands and knees, straighten your right leg and bring it up next to your right hand, with your right foot flat on the floor.

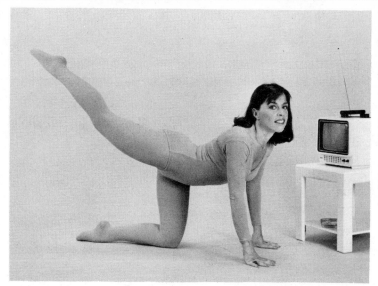

3

Continue to swing your right leg to the back and lift it as high as you can. Keep your leg straight, your foot pointed, and your hips facing the floor.

2

Raise and swing your right leg out to the side, keeping it absolutely straight.

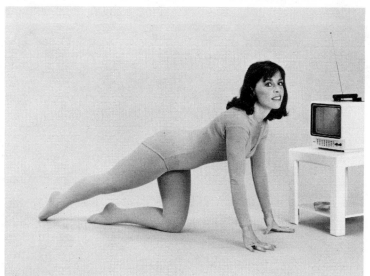

4

Without stopping, lower and lift your leg 8 times. Repeat the sequence 4 times with each leg.

BUSY LEGS

You may have to do this
exercise a few times to
establish its rhythm. Once
you do, it will become a
favorite leg workout—
especially for your thighs—
while you watch television or
listen to music.

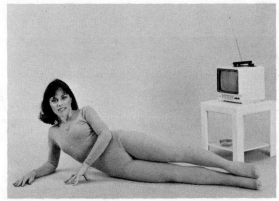

1 Lie on your right side with your
torso propped up on your elbow.
Your legs should be straight,
and your feet pointed.

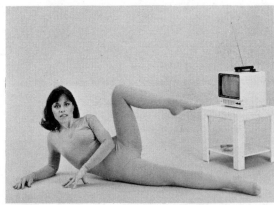

4 Bend your left knee again,
bringing it up toward your
shoulder. Your knee should face
upward.

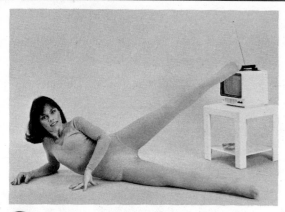

2 Raise and lower your left leg 4 times, keeping both legs straight.

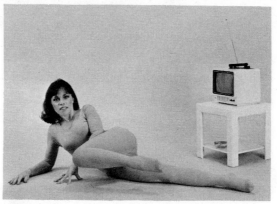

3 Bend your left leg, bringing the knee as close to your chest as you can. Bend and straighten your leg 4 times.

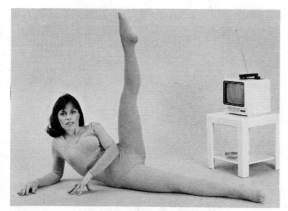

5 Straighten your left leg so it is perpendicular to your body.

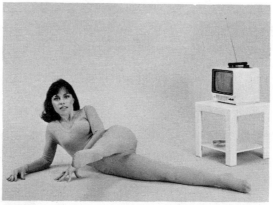

6 Lower your leg in front of your stomach, then raise and lower your left leg 4 times. Repeat the sequence 4 times with each leg.

SIDE STRETCH AND FORWARD BOUNCE

Watch television and exercise your waist and midriff! Keep your stomach muscles tightened, your bounces smooth, and focus on the screen.

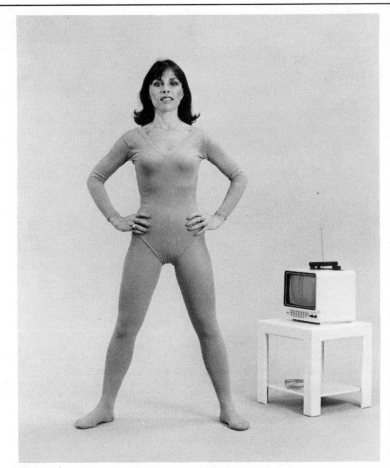

1 Stand straight with your feet apart and your hands on your hips.

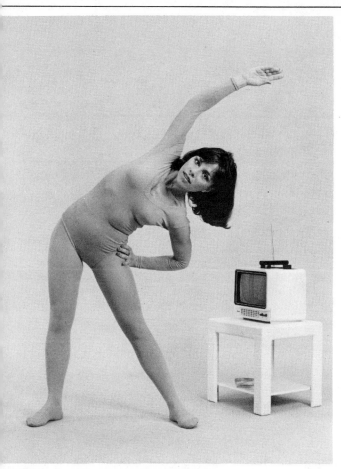

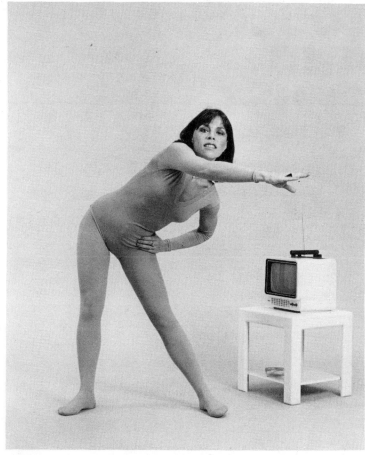

2 Curve your body to the left without bending forward or arching your back. Reach as far to the left as you can with your right arm. Bounce to the left 4 times, stretching from the waist.

3 Bending from the waist, reach forward and to the left. Bounce 4 times. Repeat the sequence to the right.

TOUCH AND TWIST

In this waist, midriff, and stomach exercise, be sure to keep your arms and legs straight—for an effective stretch in the upper arms and backs of legs.

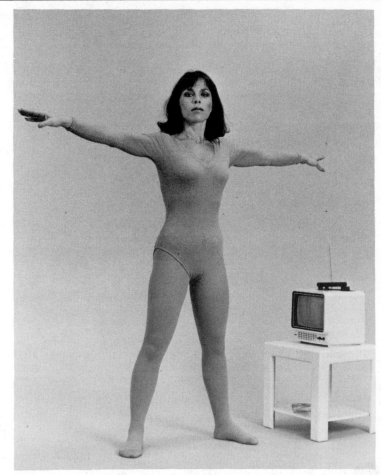

1 Stand straight with your legs apart and your arms stretched out at shoulder level.

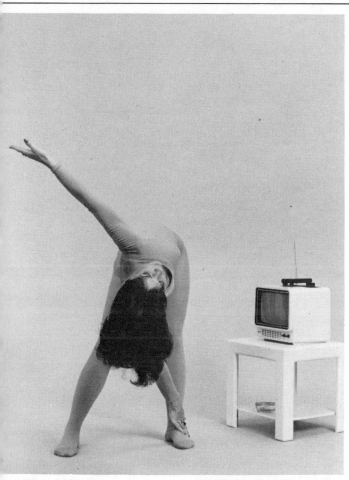

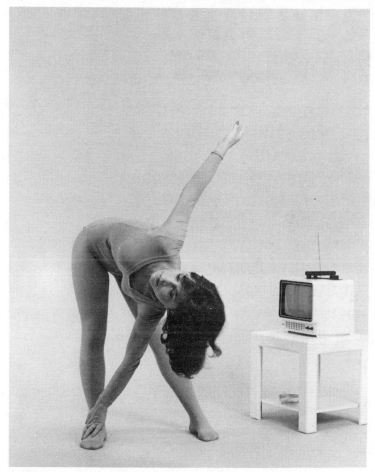

2 Bend forward at the hips. Touch your left foot with your right hand and raise your left arm in the air.

3 Twist your torso to the right, raising your right arm in the air and touching your right foot with your left hand. Twist to the left and right, touching hands to opposite feet, 8 times.

RUNNING IN PLACE

You can jog—or run—in place and get results. Although a cardiovascular exercise, this one is very good for increasing overall stamina and for toning and strengthening your legs. Slowly build up your running time to five minutes. After running in place, be sure to stretch out your legs to prevent stiffness.

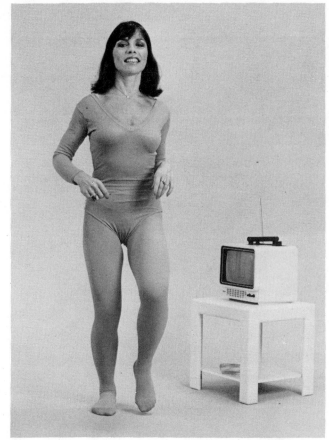

1 Run in place, with your knees slightly bent and your arms relaxed. Starting with 30 seconds of running, work up to 4 or 5 minutes. Be sure your heels touch the floor with each step.

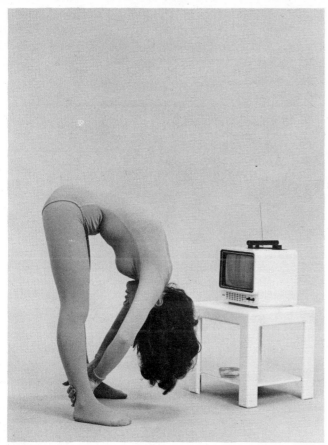

2 Stand with your feet slightly apart and your legs straight. Bend forward at the hips and clasp the backs of your ankles with your hands.

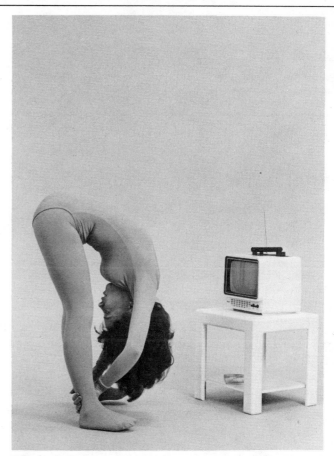

3 Keeping your knees straight, slowly pull your head and torso in as far as you can toward your legs. Hold for 4 seconds and release.

IN THE TUB

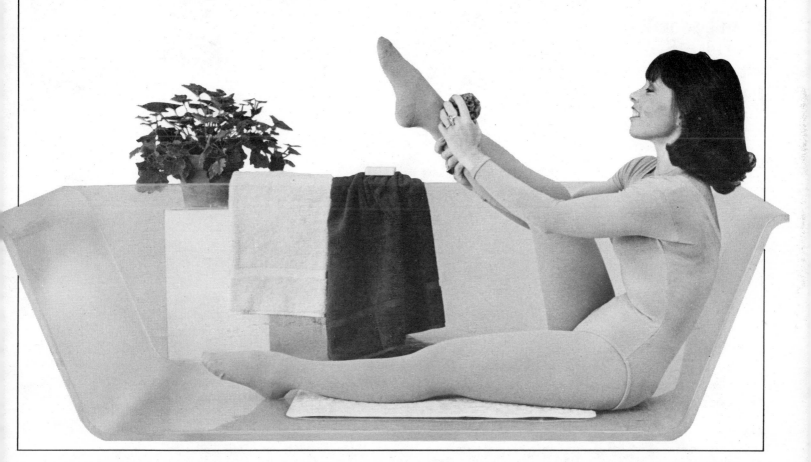

TUB LEG CIRCLES

This is an ideal tub exercise for the legs, although it can be done sitting on any surface. Stretch your legs from the hips and feel them work against the water as you make the circles.

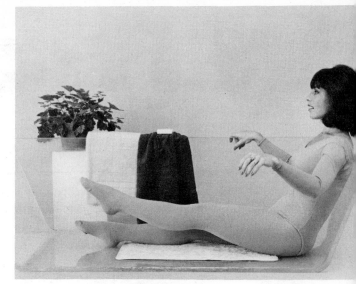

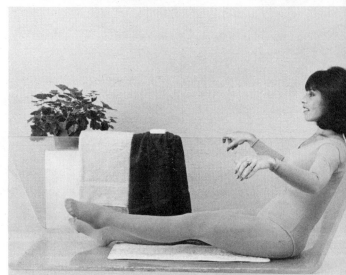

1

Sit in the tub with your legs stretched straight in front of you and your hands holding the rim of the tub. Lift your left leg about 8 inches from the tub floor. Your feet should be pointed and your stomach muscles tightened.

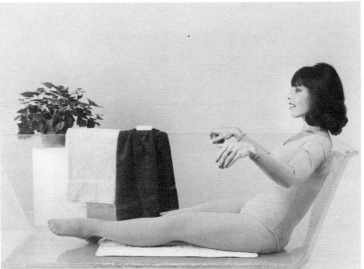

2

Keeping your legs straight, make 6 counterclockwise circles with your left leg.

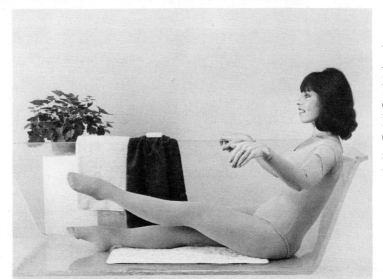

3

In the same manner, make 6 clockwise circles with your left leg.

4

Without lowering your leg, turn it so your left knee faces outward. Raise and lower your left leg 6 times. Repeat the sequence with your other leg.

FIGURE 8s

You *can* do this exercise anywhere, but muscles will tone
more quickly if you save it for
the tub, where your legs can
work against the water.
Make slow, steady turns with
each leg.

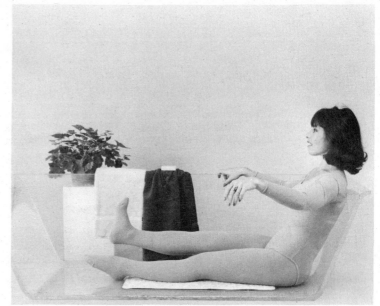

1 Sit in the tub with your legs
straight in front of you and your
hands holding the rim of the
tub. Raise your right leg several
inches higher than your left leg
and flex your right foot. Your
left foot should be pointed.

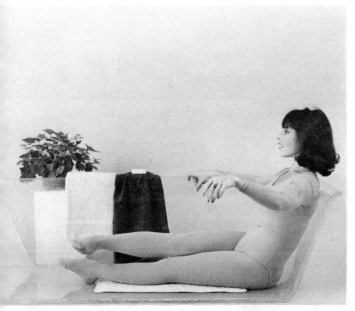

2 Keeping your right leg straight and foot flexed, make a figure 8, beginning by turning your toes to the left . . .

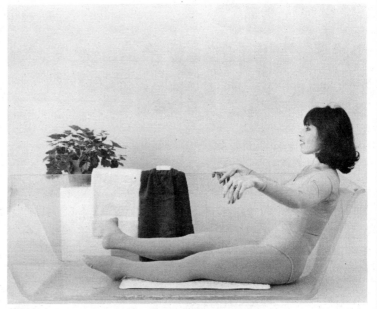

3 . . . then to the right, as you cross your right leg over your left leg. Make 6 complete figure 8s in this manner. Repeat the sequence with your other leg.

SIT-UP WITHOUT SPLASHING

Relaxing in the tub may be one of the most enjoyable things you can do for yourself all day. However, take a few minutes and give your stomach muscles a workout. This exercise also strengthens your lower back and tones inner thighs.

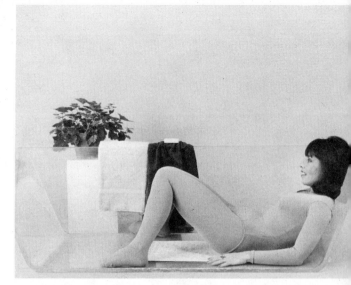

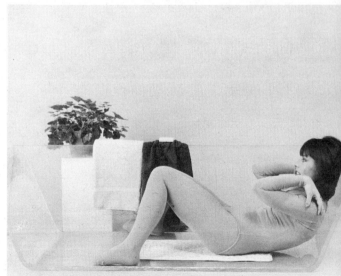

1

Sit in the tub with your knees bent and pressed together, feet pressing against the tub walls, and arms resting at your sides. Your lower back should be flat on the tub floor, with your upper back leaning against the back of the tub.

2

Keeping your head above water, place the palms of your hands on your shoulders.

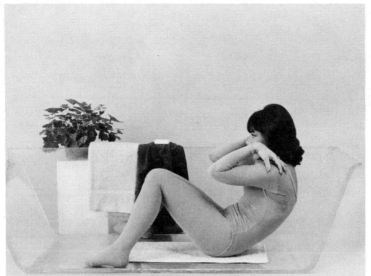

3

Slowly bring your torso up to a sitting position with your back rounded. Hold this three-quarter position for 3 seconds.

4

When you reach a full sitting position, straighten your back, keeping your stomach muscles pulled in and your feet pressing against the tub sides. Round your back and slowly lower your torso to the tub floor. Repeat the sequence 4 times.

SHOWER STRETCH

This gentle stretch is perfect for the shower. If done in the morning, it wakes up the body and works out any muscle kinks. At the end of the day, it helps release built-up tension and muscle strain.

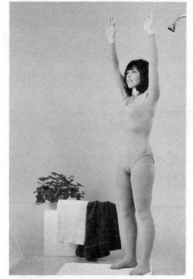

1

Stand straight with feet slightly apart and arms raised above your head. Keep your stomach and buttocks muscles tightened.

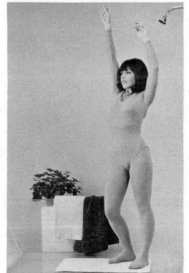

2

Keeping your left leg straight, bend your right knee slightly, and stretch your right arm over your head.

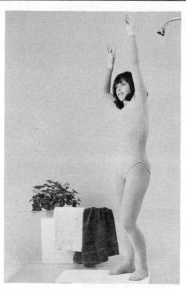

3

In the same manner, straighten your right leg, bend your left knee, and stretch your left arm over your head. Bend your knees and stretch, alternating sides, 6 times.

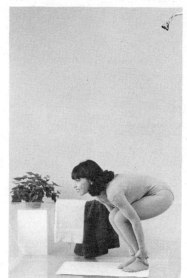

5

With your feet flat on the tub floor, bend your knees and clasp both ankles with your hands. Keep your back straight and your head up. Hold for 3 seconds.

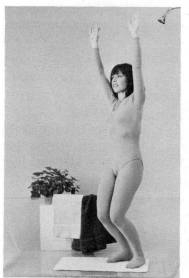

4

While stretching both arms over your head, bend your knees and lower your torso as far as you can, keeping your heels flat on the tub floor. Bend and straighten your knees and stretch 4 times.

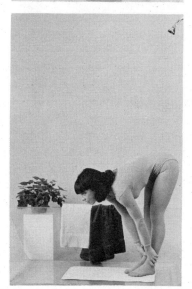

6

Holding onto your ankles, slowly straighten your legs, lifting your buttocks in the air. Hold for 3 seconds. Repeat the sequence 4 times.

DRY AND TWIST

After a bath or shower, muscles are warm, supple, and ready for exercise. Turn drying off into a small but effective workout for your arms, waist, and midriff. Keep your stomach muscles tightened.

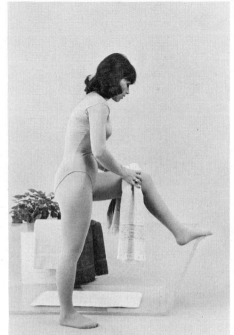

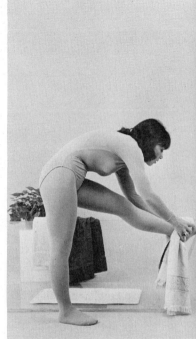

1 Stand straight with your left foot resting on the rim of the tub. Hold the towel in both hands and place it above your left knee.

2 In one continuous motion, bend your torso at the hips and straighten your left leg and arms, as you stretch forward to dry your lower leg. Bend and straighten each leg 6 times.

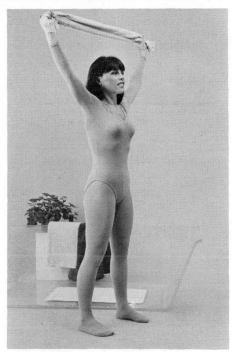

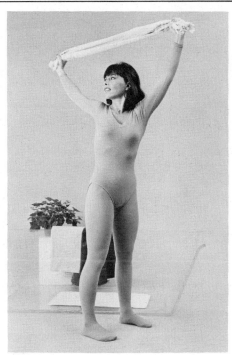

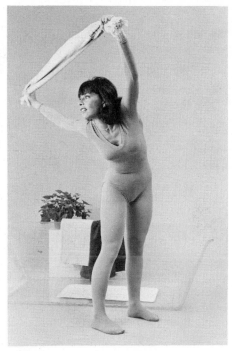

3 Stand straight with your feet slightly apart, holding the towel taut over your head. Your arms should be straight.

4 Keeping your arms and legs straight, twist your torso as far to the right as you can.

5 Without moving your hips and legs, bend at the waist. Twist and bend to the left and right, alternating, 6 times.

BACK TOWEL WIPE

Don't just dry your back. Use that time to exercise your upper arms, and—in Step 4— your hips, where you can pretend you are doing the Twist.

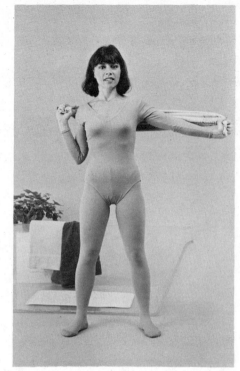

1 Stand straight with your legs about 12 inches apart. Hold the towel in both hands and place it across your upper back. Pull the towel back and forth, moving it up and down your back, 6 times.

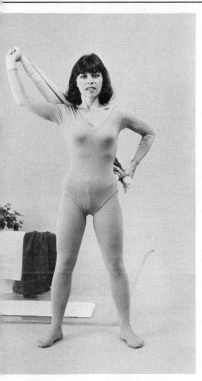

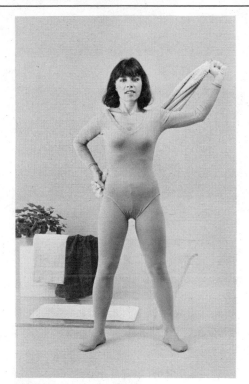

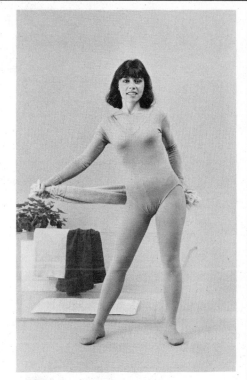

2 Hold the towel diagonally across your back. Pull the towel up and down 6 times.

3 Reverse the diagonal and pull the towel up and down 6 times.

4 Stretch the towel across your buttocks. As you pull the towel back and forth 6 times, push your hips from side to side, while shifting your weight.

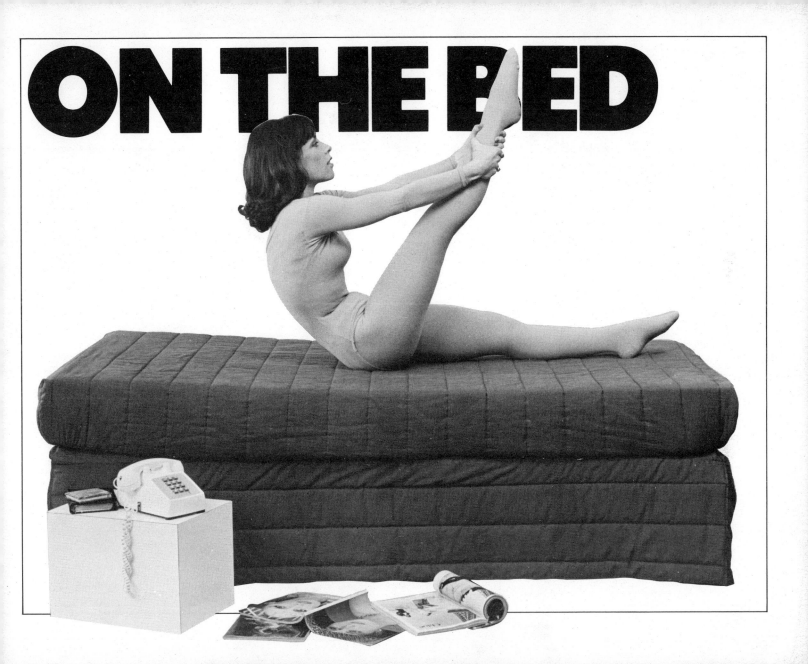

SUPINE STRETCH

A workout with a dual purpose. If done in the morning, this easy stretch awakens your body muscles slowly and readies them for a busy day. At bed time, it releases built-up tension in your muscles and relaxes your body for sleep.

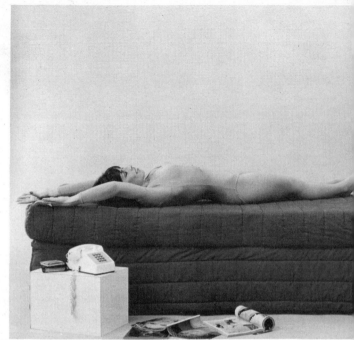

1 Lie on your back, legs straight and feet pointed, with your arms stretched out on the bed behind your head. Keeping your body flat, stretch your left arm and your left leg. Your right side should be relaxed. Hold for 3 seconds.

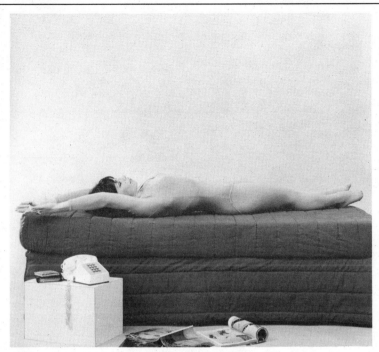

2 In the same manner, stretch your right arm and your right leg. Hold for 3 seconds.

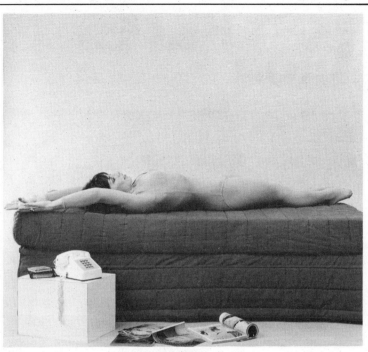

3 Stretch both arms and legs and tighten the muscles in your entire body. Hold for 3 seconds, then relax. Repeat the sequence as often as you wish.

BENT KNEE DROP

This is one exercise that can be done on any flat surface—bed, floor, or beach. Keep your back flat and your stomach muscles tightened, as you try to reach the surface with the knee of your working leg.

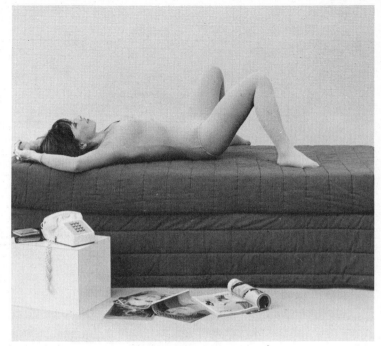

1 Lie on your back, elbows bent and hands clasped above your head. Your knees should be bent and as far apart as possible.

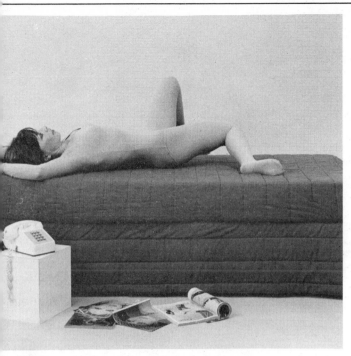 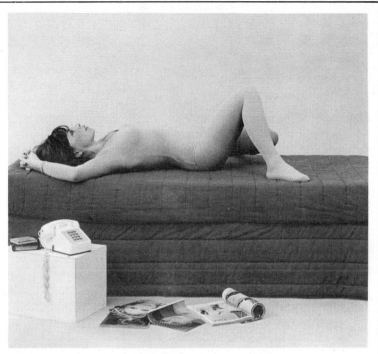

2 Keeping your back flat on the bed and your stomach muscles tightened, lower your right knee as far to the inside as you can without lifting your buttocks off the bed. Feel the stretch in your thigh.

3 In the same manner, lower your left thigh. Repeat the sequence as often as you wish.

SIT-UP AND LEG STRETCH

This exercise combines a sit-up with a leg stretch to give your stomach, back, and legs a full workout. Keep your movements and stretches slow and smooth, whether you do them on a soft bed or a hard surface.

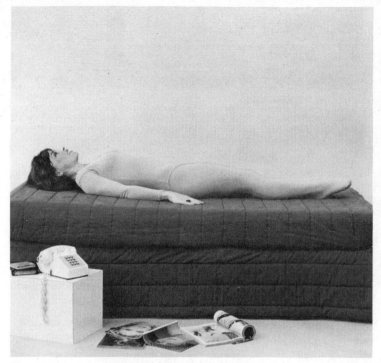

1 Lie on your back, legs straight, feet pointed, and arms resting at your sides.

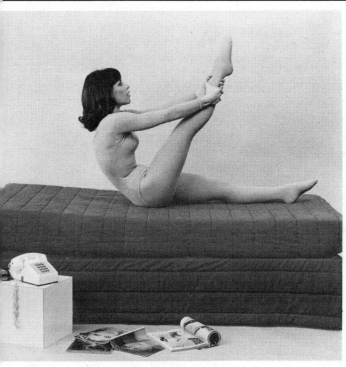

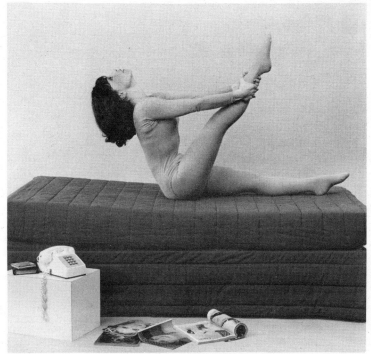

2 In one continuous motion, swing your arms up and raise your right leg, clasping it at the ankle with both hands. Your leg must remain straight and your back should be rounded. Hold for 3 seconds.

3 Slowly straighten your back and lift your chin to the ceiling. Be sure your stomach muscles are tightened. Hold for 3 seconds. Return to the original position and repeat Steps 2 and 3 with your left leg. Repeat the sequence 6 times.

BED BICYCLE

This may be one of the most common but effective stomach exercises. So why not do it in bed, while deciding what to wear—or while waiting for the bath-room. Be sure to stretch out your legs and push with your feet when cycling.

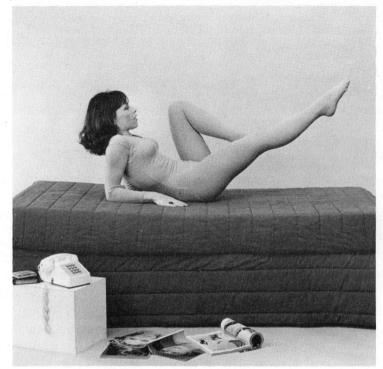

1 Lie on the bed with your torso propped up on your elbows. Your right leg should be straight and at a 45-degree angle with the bed, with your left leg raised and bent at the knee.

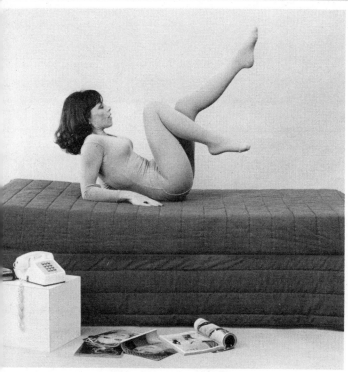

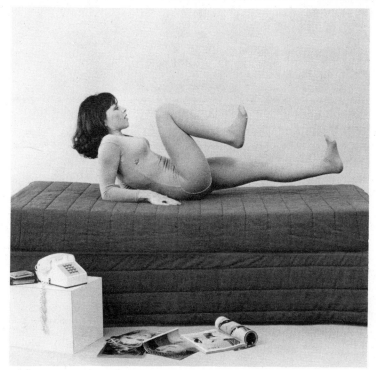

2 With pointed feet, slowly move your legs as if you were bicycling. Make the pedaling motions 8 times with each leg.

3 Flex your feet and make 8 cycling motions with each leg. Repeat the sequence 4 times.

HUG AND STRETCH

This exercise for your stomach and legs is easier to do on a bed than on a hard surface. Keep your shoulders off the bed, your stomach muscles tightened, and your feet pointed. When you repeat Steps 3 through 6, try to develop a slow, steady rhythm.

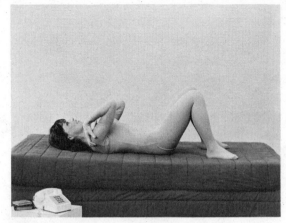

1 Lie on your back, knees bent, feet flat on the bed and your palms on your shoulders.

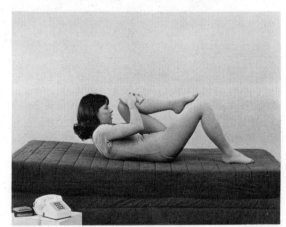

4 Reverse legs and hug your left knee to your chest.

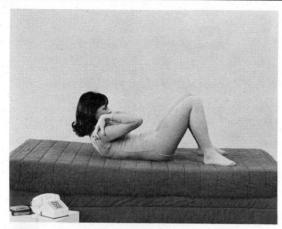

2 Lift your head and shoulders off the bed. Hold for 3 seconds.

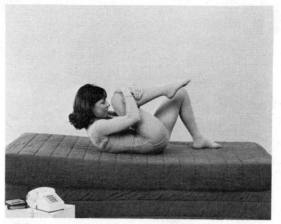

3 Without lowering your shoulders, hug your right knee to your chest.

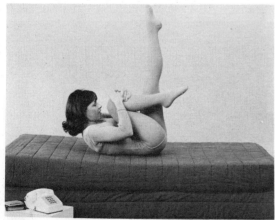

5 In one continuous motion, hug your right knee to your chest, and straighten your left leg.

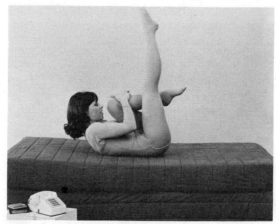

6 In the same manner, hug your left leg. Repeat Steps 3-6 at least 4 times.

ON-THE-BED SCISSORS

Do this exercise every morning *before* you get up or every night *before* you go to sleep. Or while watching television. It is one of the best workouts for toning and firming inner and outer thighs.

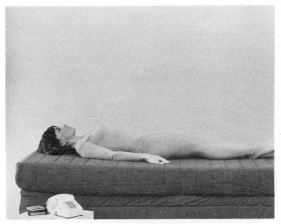

1 Lie on your back, legs straight and feet pointed, with your arms resting at your sides.

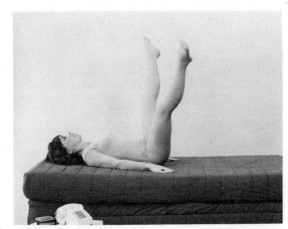

4 Open your legs as wide as you can, keeping your feet pointed.

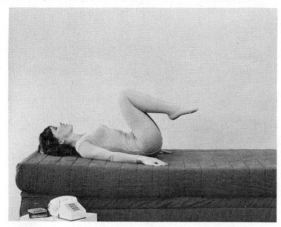

2 Bend your legs and bring them to your chest.

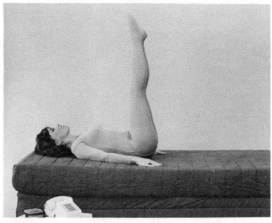

3 Straighten your legs so that they are perpendicular to the bed. Keep your feet pointed.

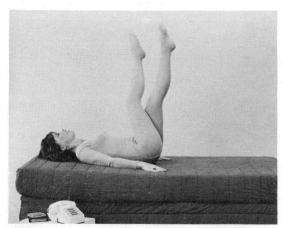

5 Bring your legs together in scissor fashion. Open and cross your legs, alternating, 16 times.

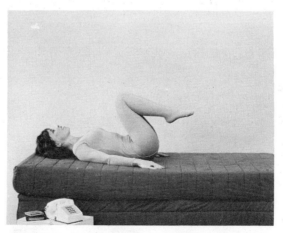

6 Bend your knees and slowly lower your legs, so your feet are flat on the bed.

BACK BOUNCES

A flexible back and flexible legs are healthy ones. This back and leg exercise for the bed—or floor, if you're watching television or playing with children—is one of the best. Keep your bounces slow and smooth. It is also an effective workout for your inner thighs, if you bring your feet as close to your body as you can.

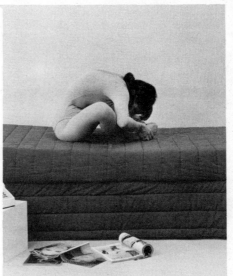

1

Sit on the bed with your feet pressed together and your heels as close to your body as possible. Clasp your ankles with your hands and, round your back. Bring your forehead to your feet. Gently bounce from the hips 8 times.

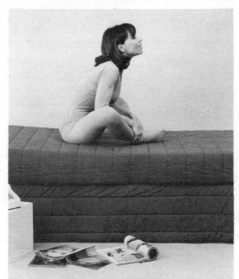

2

Straighten your back and bring your elbows inside your legs to press on your knees. Gently bounce 8 times from the hips, keeping your back straight and your head up.

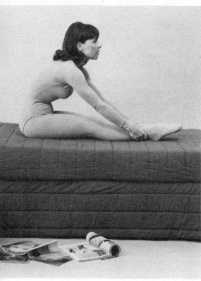

3

Extend your legs in front of you and point your feet. Straighten your arms and clasp your ankles with both hands. Your back should be rounded and your feet pointed.

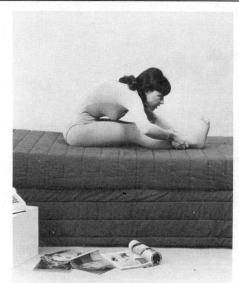

5

Flex your feet and bounce another 8 times.

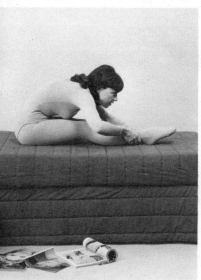

4

Bring your torso as close to your legs as you can and bounce 8 times, keeping your head up.

CAT STRETCH

Another exercise that is perfect for waking up the body in the morning or for relaxing it before sleep. Do it slowly and enjoy the stretch. Keep stomach muscles tightened for added toning benefits.

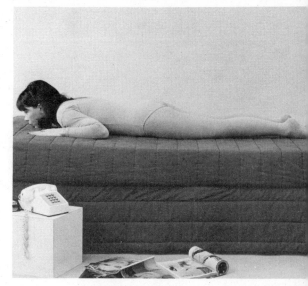

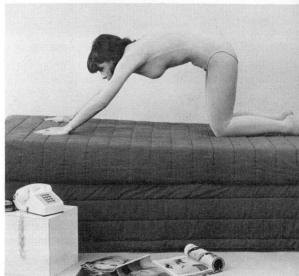

1

Lie on your stomach, with legs straight and chin resting on the bed. Bend your elbows and keep your arms close to your torso.

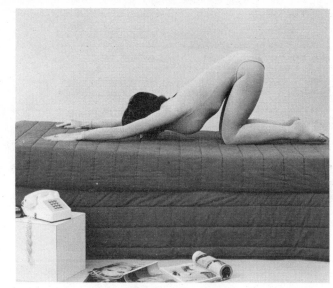

2

Slowly straighten your arms and lift up off the bed. Round your back slightly and tighten your stomach muscles.

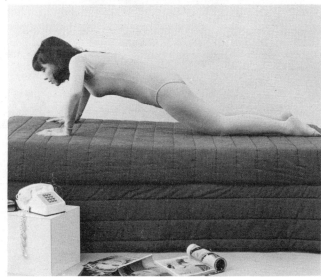

3

Keeping your palms flat on the bed and your arms straight, lower your upper torso and face to the bed. Your back should be straight and your buttocks in the air. Be sure your stomach muscles are tightened.

4

Bend your elbows and return to the original position. Repeat the sequence 6 times.

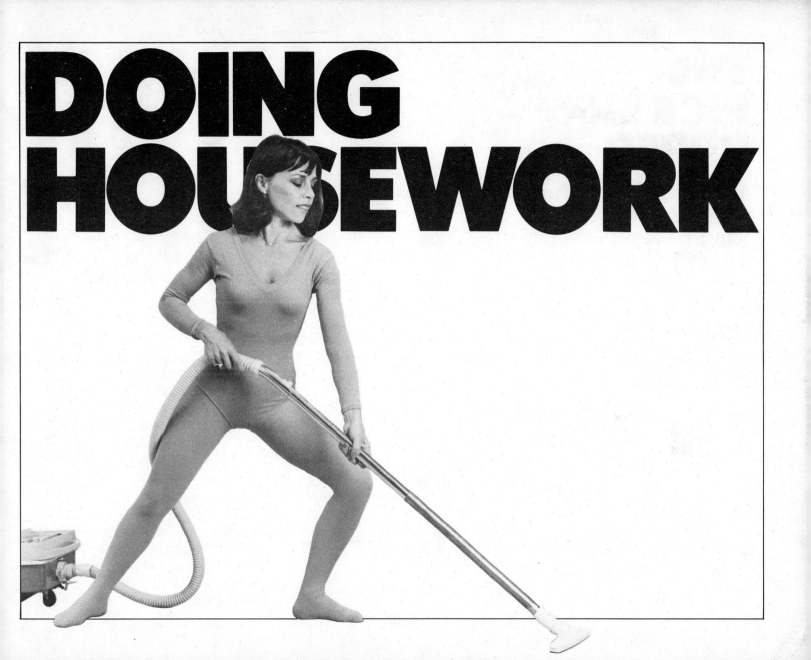

THE PICKER-UPPER

An exercise for every time you have to pick up something from the floor—or when you're looking for an object on the bottom shelf of a bookcase or cupboard. However, don't do it quickly, or if you have a bad back.

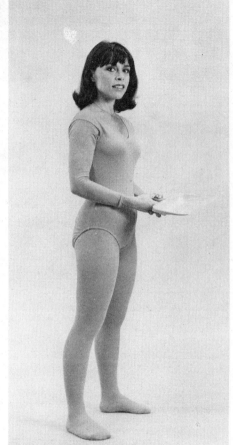

1 Stand straight with your legs apart. Your arms can be relaxed at your sides or holding onto a dust pan or cloth.

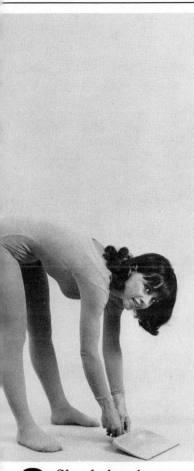

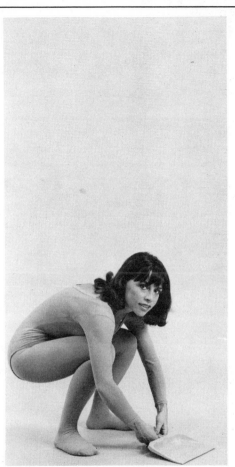

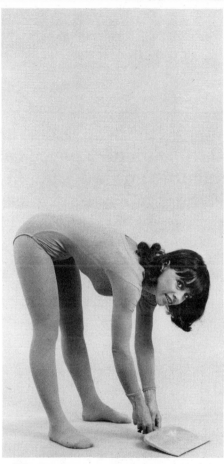

2 Slowly bend your torso forward at the hips and let your arms drop to the floor. Tighten your stomach muscles.

3 Bend your knees and squat, while you pick up something from the floor. Keep your heels flat on the floor.

4 Slowly straighten your legs and return to the original position. Repeat the sequence as often as you need.

VACUUM LUNGE

Vacuuming must be done, but now with this exercise and the one following, you can vacuum and work out at the same time! This exercise is particularly good for your legs and buttocks.

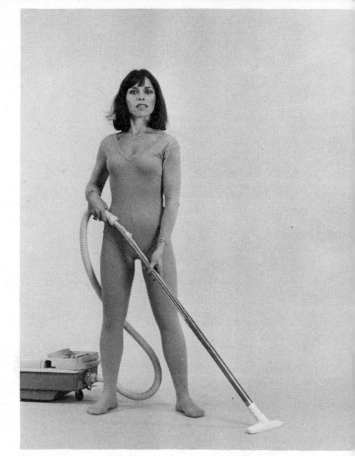

1 Standing straight with your feet apart, hold onto the handle of the vacuum cleaner with both hands.

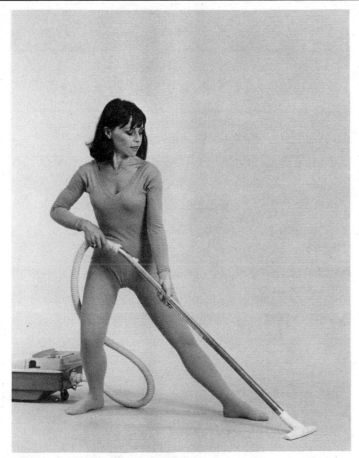

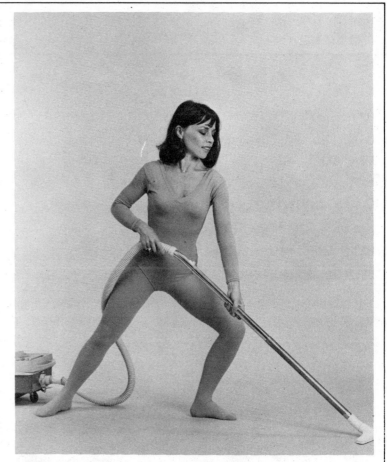

2 Slightly bend your right knee, leaning your weight on the outside of your right foot. Your left foot should be turned out and your left leg stretched out. Keep your body facing outward.

3 Without moving your feet, bend forward on your left knee and stretch out your right leg. Lunge forward and back 4 times with each leg.

CLEAN SWEEP

You can work your stomach and back muscles while you vacuum, sweep, or mop, if you make this exercise part of your cleaning routine. If you keep your legs perfectly straight, they will benefit from the gentle stretch.

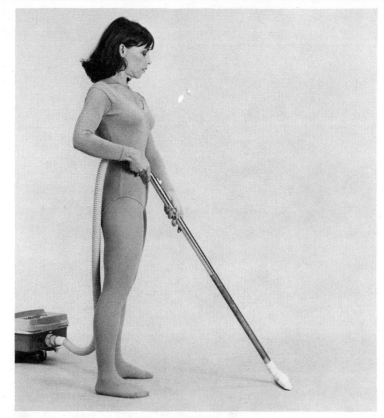

1 Stand straight with your feet slightly apart. Hold onto the vacuum cleaner handle with both hands.

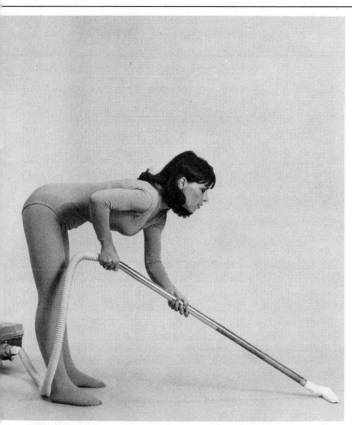

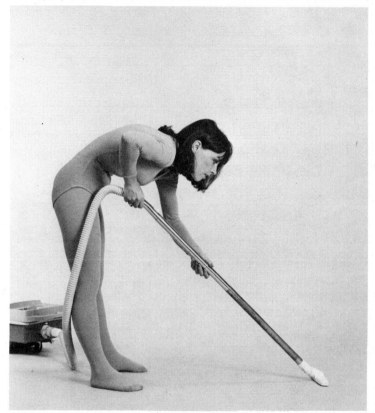

2 Keeping your legs straight, bend forward at the hips until your torso is parallel to the floor. Be sure your back is straight, your head up, and your stomach muscles tightened.

3 Slowly round your back as you bring the vacuum cleaner toward you. Continue to flatten and round your back as you vacuum.

SWEEP AND TWIST

It may take a few more minutes to sweep with this exercise, but the workout it gives your waist is worth it. Do not let your hips move when you reach back with the broom. Once you become accustomed to these movements, you can do this twist without a broom.

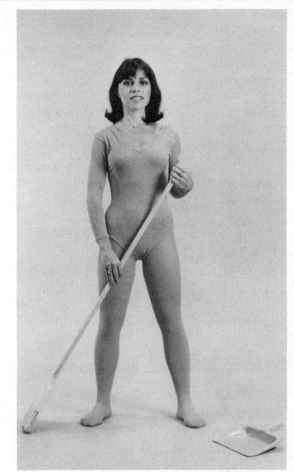

1 Stand straight with your legs apart and your hands holding the broom.

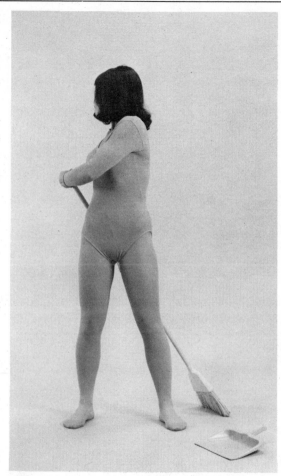

2 Keeping your hips still and facing forward, twist as far to the right as you can.

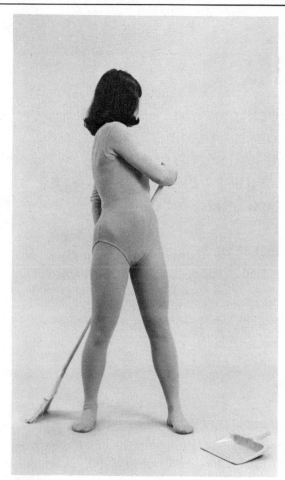

3 In the same manner, twist to the left. Repeat until the surface is completely swept.

THE DUSTER

Yes, you can exercise as you dust, wash, or polish a table —and even when you scrub a floor or rinse off walls! This mini-workout is excellent for toning the upper arms and for releasing tension in the upper back and shoulders.

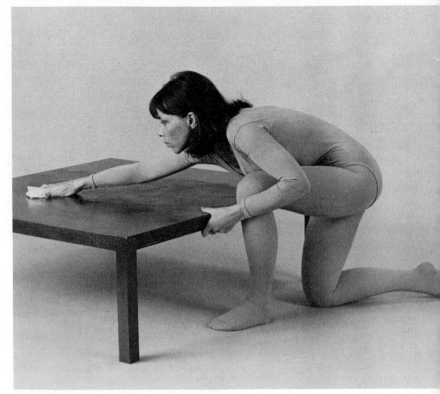

1 Stand straight with your legs together or kneel on one knee near the table to be dusted. With a straight arm, make 4 wide clockwise circles, then 4 wide counterclockwise circles.

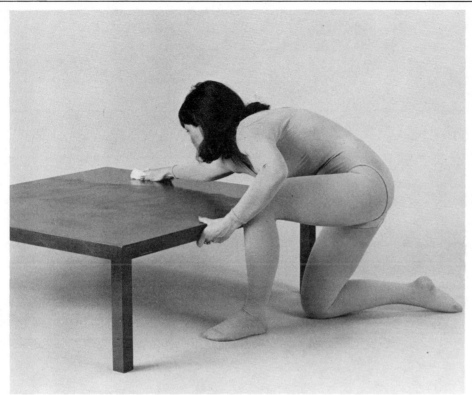

2 Keeping your arm straight, move it from side to side 4 times, or until the surface is completely dusted.

DUST AWAY

Although shown standing, this exercise can also be done on your hands and knees. Whether done standing or kneeling, it helps firm and tone stomach muscles and upper arms; if done standing, it also stretches the backs of your legs. Either way, keep your stomach muscles tightened.

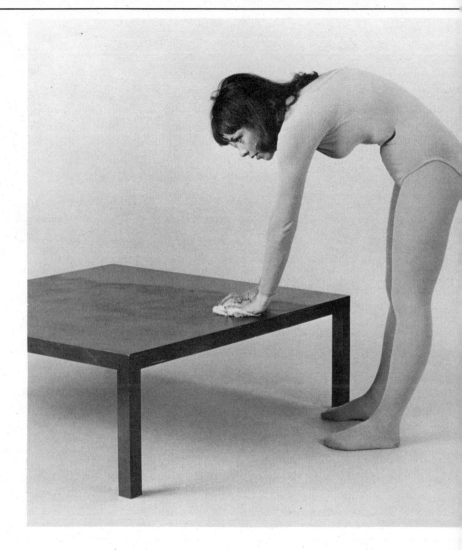

1

Stand with your legs straight and your feet slightly apart. Bend your torso forward from the hips and round your back. Your arms should be straight and your hands placed on the table, holding a dust cloth.

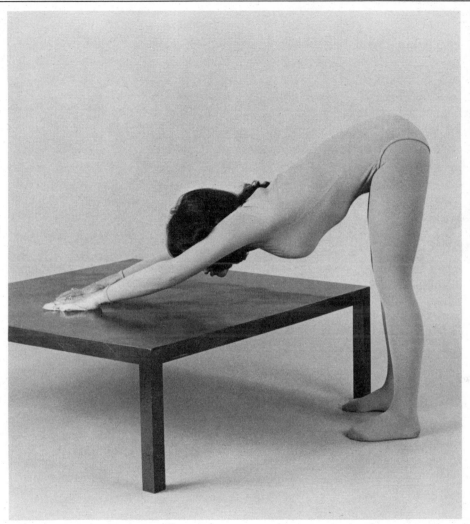

2

Keeping your arms straight, slowly move them forward, stretching from the hips. Your back should be straight and your stomach muscles tightened. Round and straighten your back until the surface is dusted.

HEELS OFF

This simple exercise can be done while washing dishes, if you stand on a phone book, or by stopping on stairs as you go from one floor to another. It keeps the backs of the legs, especially the ankle and calf area, stretched and flexible. Women who wear heels and men and women who jog or walk long distances should do this exercise daily.

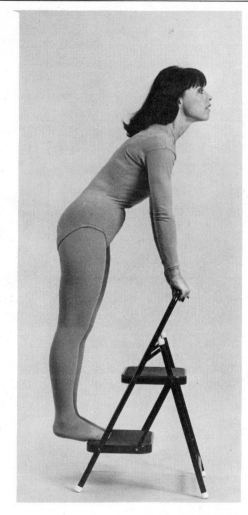

1

Stand straight on a ladder or on a thick book such as a dictionary or phone book. Only the balls of your feet (not your heels) should be supported by the ladder or book.

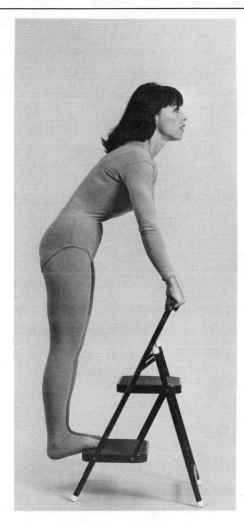

2
Lower your heels as far toward the floor as you comfortably can. Hold the lowered position for 8 seconds.

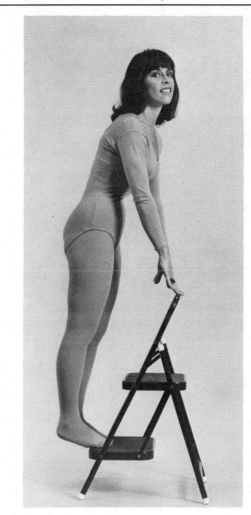

3
Lift your heels as high as you can, keeping the balls of your feet flat on the ladder or book. Repeat the sequence as often as you wish.

CABINET-REACHER

Each time you reach for something in the kitchen, bathroom, or office, take the opportunity to do this stretch. It's an easy workout for the buttocks. For additional toning, bounce your raised leg, but remember to keep your buttock muscles tightened.

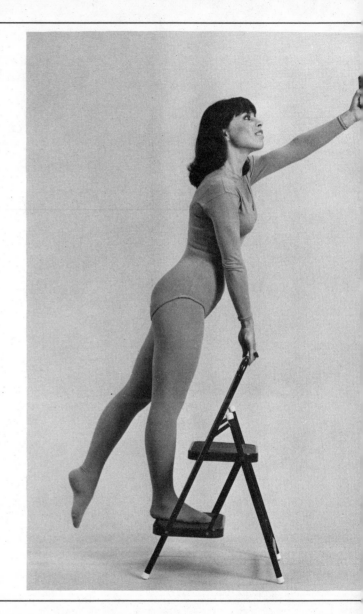

1

Stand on the floor or on a step ladder. Hold onto the ladder or a counter, if possible. In one continuous motion, reach with a straight arm for the item needed, and stretch your leg straight out behind you.

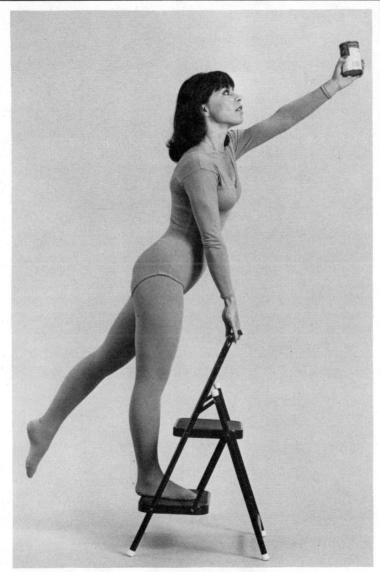

2

Lift your leg higher and hold for 3 seconds. Be sure your stomach and buttock muscles are tightened. Change sides and repeat the sequence.